"Conversations with colleagues characterized by candor and vulnerability lay the foundation for trust-filled and supportive peer connections. These thoughtful, powerful, and authentic real-life stories can serve as the foundation for enduring resilience, healing, and culture change. This will make a difference for the good."

**Stephen Swensen**, MD, *author of* Mayo Clinic Strategies to Reduce Burnout: 12 Actions to Create the Ideal Workplace, *former director of Leadership and Organization Development, Mayo Clinic, professor emeritus, Mayo Clinic College of Medicine and Science*

"Much more than wellness lectures, pizza parties, or research reports, stories have a unique way of helping us feel seen and less alone. This is particularly needed in healthcare, where we look around and think everyone else is 'fine' because of a culture of stigma and silence. This book is not only grounded in our narratives, but it also helps teach through them, and that combination is unique and needed."

**Jessi Gold**, MD, MS, *chief wellness officer of the University of Tennessee System and author of* How Do You Feel?

"This book is an extraordinarily moving compilation of stories told by courageous, caring and very human physicians. Accounts of struggle, growth and resilience illuminate the complex inner lives of doctors as they navigate work, family, health and personal challenges. The facilitator guide offers a practical roadmap for using these stories to build community and connection through discussion groups and workshops. I highly recommend this book to physicians, to those who work with or care about physicians, and to anyone seeking to better understand the complex experience of people working in health care today."

**Susannah Rowe**, MD, MPH, FACS, *associate chief medical officer for Wellness and Professional Vitality, Boston Medical Center*

"Stories frame our experience. They also inform our personal and collective journeys of healing and wellbeing. This book's collection of authentic narratives is a vital resource for all physicians, whether in training or in practice."

**Mark F. Carroll**, MD, FAAP, *chief medical officer, Blue Cross Blue Shield of Arizona Medicaid Plans*

# Physician Wellness and Resilience

*Physician Wellness and Resilience: Narrative Prompts to Address Burnout* explores 26 compelling narratives from practicing doctors and medical students as they share their personal and professional encounters in their own words.

This volume seeks to expand the conversations around burnout and mental health in the medical profession and advocates for a deeper appreciation of physicians as human beings, complete with a range of emotions and fallibilities. Its diverse array of professionals spans various medical specialties and career stages and covers a range of experiences, including dealing with sexism, committing medical errors, handling challenging colleagues, and the fear and commitment involved in treating patients with COVID-19. Chapters include discussion prompts to encourage creative problem-solving among readers and nurture a caring and supportive work environment for physicians seeking assistance.

Designed for use in medical school seminars and physician wellness seminars, this book is essential reading for physicians, junior doctors, medical students, and mental health professionals who work with these populations.

**Pauline Davies** is Professor of Practice and teaches human communication at Arizona State University. Specializing in cancer research outreach, she is also an award-winning former BBC science and health broadcaster.

**Dr Cynthia M. Stonnington** is an award-winning psychiatrist, educator, and wellness expert at the Mayo Clinic in Arizona. She directed the psychiatry and psychology department for ten years.

# Routledge Focus on Mental Health

Routledge Focus on Mental Health presents short books on current topics, linking in with cutting-edge research and practice.

**Titles in the series:**

For a full list of titles in this series, please visit https://www.routledge.com/Routledge-Focus-on-Mental-Health/book-series/RFMH

# Physician Wellness and Resilience

## Narrative Prompts to Address Burnout

**Edited by
Pauline Davies and
Cynthia M. Stonnington**

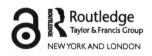

Routledge
Taylor & Francis Group

NEW YORK AND LONDON

ISBN: 978-1-032-73829-1 (hbk)
ISBN: 978-1-032-75681-3 (pbk)
ISBN: 978-1-003-47517-0 (ebk)

DOI: 10.4324/9781003475170

Typeset in Times New Roman
by codeMantra

*This book is dedicated to all those healthcare professionals who were brave enough to share their story for the benefit of others.*

# Contents

# Preface

Not long before COVID-19 struck, Dr Cynthia Stonnington, then Chair of Psychiatry and Psychology at the Mayo Clinic in Arizona, met with Professor Pauline Davies from the Hugh Downs School of Human Communication at Arizona State University and they conceived of a project to help doctors in trouble.

Cynthia works at the sharp end of the medical profession, dealing daily with crises experienced by her colleagues. Pauline was taken aback to discover that physicians worldwide were grappling with burnout and mental issues, in some cases leading to the abandonment of their careers. The appalling attrition rate is not only a human tragedy but also a waste of valuable resources that the world can ill afford. The acute psychological problems many physicians face stem from a combination of a high-stress work environment, fear of failure, and a deep reluctance to share their emotions and experiences with fellow professionals. In many cases, they labor under the misconception that their medical license will be withdrawn if they admit a need for mental healthcare. Efforts to remove mental health questions from licensure and credentialing applications and establish confidential support systems for physicians seeking help are certainly a step in the right direction. But there remains the fundamental problem of an extremely demanding culture and a system that imposes barriers to help-seeking.

Pauline and Cynthia made the decision to conduct candid interviews with a couple of dozen physicians and medical students from various specialties, systems, and regions. Doctors and students were invited to share the problems and the joys that they encountered throughout their careers. All the stories are deeply moving, inspiring, and informative; recounting them proved an emotional journey for some, often reducing both the interviewer and interviewee to tears. Yet, they provide a glimpse into the complexities of human nature, including our capacity for generosity, personal forgiveness, and psychological healing within the critical arena of medical practice. The resulting compilation of narratives holds valuable lessons for physician training and well-being. It is our hope that by reading, reflecting on, and discussing these accounts, medical students and early career physicians will understand the challenges faced by members of the medical profession, appreciate the rewards offered by a career in medicine, and find solace in the knowledge that they are not alone. Within the medical community, a remarkable group of individuals devotes themselves not for financial gain, but because they genuinely care!

What follows are the words of the doctors and medical students themselves—words imbued with grace and compassion.

Each story is compelling and genuine. The interviews have been lightly edited for clarity. To protect the anonymity of the participants, their names and other identifying details have been altered. All individuals involved willingly agreed to share their stories, and the project was approved by the Mayo Clinic Institutional Review Board.

We extend our heartfelt gratitude to all those who bravely shared their traumatic or challenging experiences, entrusting us to relay their valuable lessons to the wider community.

# Acknowledgments

We received valuable assistance in completing this book from Olivia Zeitlin, and wish to thank Professors Jennifer Linde and Linda Lederman and video editor Edward (Bill) Bedrava for helping to produce a film compilation of the stories. Finally, our life partners, Jim Weinstein and Paul Davies, deserve thanks too. The interviews were conducted with grant assistance from the Mayo Clinic.

Pauline Davies
Professor of Practice, Hugh Downs School of Human Communication,
Arizona State University
Cynthia M. Stonnington, MD
Professor of Psychiatry, Mayo Clinic College of Medicine and Science

# How to Use the Stories in This Book

Like their patients, doctors experience and suffer the vicissitudes of life. The true stories in this book are intended to promote well-being and cultivate a supportive and caring community within the medical profession. All contributors gave written consent to publish their stories under pseudonyms. Their stories were transcribed from an interview and minimally edited. They are meant to be raw, rather than polished essays. Readers are prompted to reflect on their own similar experiences, or put themselves in the narrator's shoes. The stories are meant to inspire medical professionals and students to seek help when needed and collectively work toward a fulfilling medical practice, where each person feels valued and capable of caring for themselves in addition to their patients.

If using in a workshop setting, we suggest the following:

1 Consider roughly 60 minutes for the workshop, potentially part of a weekly, monthly, or quarterly series. For each session, pick one or two stories (depending on the length of the story) covering the themes that seem most relevant to your group. Ideally, a facilitator coordinates the sessions and discussions.

2 Set ground rules at the beginning of the session to ensure confidentiality and mutual respect.

3 Participants take turns reading each paragraph of the story out loud. Alternatively, individuals can read the whole story silently; however, reading aloud serves to focus attention and increase engagement.

4 Divide into groups of 4–10 people and discuss the story. Each person chooses a prompt. Take 5–10 minutes for individuals to write their responses. Then participants volunteer to share reflections with each other and discuss, or depending on the size, reconvene in the large group.

5 We encourage facilitators to direct users to the bibliography at the back of the book for a list of useful resources and references. Some of the reading materials or videos are suitable for use within the session. If so inclined, consider pairing stories with relevant quotes from literature, e.g., novels, poetry, for further inspiration. A few examples of relevant novels are listed in the bibliography. Ideally, facilitators will also provide local or institutional resources for mental health and peer support.

# Part I

# Student Life

# 1 Insight

*Kelsey Zhang is a restaurant enthusiast and MD-PhD student who has completed her third year of medical school and is working on her doctoral research. Medical school has been very tough. She's struggled juggling academic, family, cultural and social pressures, unrealized culinary ambitions, and mental illness. Fortunately, aided by her friends and colleagues, alongside psychotherapy and medication, she has gained insight and the ability to get through her hardest times.*

I am a Chinese American. I grew up with parents who always wanted me to become a doctor, and I thought I wanted this too. I did undergraduate at a liberal arts college where I was a pre-med double-degree piano and neuroscience major. During that time, I got very involved with the co-op system, cooking for a large number of people. At that point, I wanted to open a restaurant.

I applied to medical school in my fifth year of college, but I had a really bad MCAT score. I wasn't getting many interviews. As my back-up plan, I was like, "Well, let me try to open a restaurant and see what happens." I started planning for one, but then I got into a medical school and couldn't let the opportunity pass by.

Medical school was really hard—I'm sure it's hard for a lot of people. I was in a completely different environment, and I wasn't used to the learning style. Within the first three or four months I got depressed, but I never called it depression, because I was functioning. I was going to class, and from the outside, things looked fine.

I think most people who are struggling in medical school say, "Oh, but I really want to be a doctor so I'm going to keep going through this." I was like, "Maybe I should open up that pizza restaurant instead."

I didn't seek help until the middle of the second year. I started going to a therapist, but it was weird because I didn't even go on my own terms. I had talked to the dean, and she said, "Maybe you should go see our mental health clinician who is really good. If your performance isn't going so well in medical school, it's often some kind of testing issue. She deals with testing anxiety."

DOI: 10.4324/9781003475170-2

So I went, and within five minutes she's like, "OK, why are you really here?" She saw it was depression and how life was not working out; it wasn't just testing anxiety.

I started taking medication probably sometime late in the second year. I would take it inconsistently because I thought I was fine, that I didn't really need it because I had ups and downs.

That second year, I wanted to leave medical school, do a music therapy degree and then return later. All my advisors encouraged me to continue through third year and finish it, because that's when you get your clinical rotations and get to see which area you like.

I did do that, and I'm glad, because I found out that I really like surgery. I hadn't expected that. But now, I'm like, "I actually want to do residency. I really love doing the surgeries."

So, here I am, third year, wanting to go into surgery, which is a competitive specialty, but I didn't have the grades. I didn't know my stuff. I didn't have the Step 1 score, so there was a lot of pressure building up. At the same time, I also had to study for my neuro shelf and I was nervous about that too. But the thing that tipped me over was a meeting with one of the surgeons. He had offered me this *awesome* research opportunity. He was checking in: "Hey, how's the manuscript going?" I just looked down. I was like, "I need to go home right now." I just said it was going well but that I wasn't feeling good, and I left. I basically imploded. I couldn't manage my depression anymore and I just had to stop school.

Fortunately, one of the residents said, "I think someone should check in on her."

I got a call from the clerkship director. I was sobbing. I had to fly back to my parent's home and get help, learn how to do nothing and be OK with that.

I returned to medical school for exam time. It was weird because I had to tell the deans and administrators, "I'm not healthy enough to take this exam right now, but I'm not so sick that you should kick me out of school." I was like a dependent child.

I remember going to the occupational ed person. She said, "OK, you're depressed. You are supposed to do your surgery exam and your neuro exam now. I'm giving time and a half for those exams. Why don't you do surgery in two and a half weeks and one week after that do your neuro?"

I was like, "I don't think I can do that." For me, it was just so clear that it was impossible. But luckily the psychiatrist I'd been working with at the medical school helped me push the exams back by an appropriate amount. I naturally wanted to delay them as much as I could, but he was able to push me just enough to do them. I ended up being OK. I passed!

The people in the medical school were very helpful and I'm glad I returned. The dean gave me her cellphone number right away. I also had a very close relationship with the psychiatrist mentor. He would call and email me all the time during this period. That was great. All the people I was close with were really good.

I was terrified it would be different because a friend at another medical school had a suicide attempt that led to a lot of trouble. The school worried that since he was a harm to himself, might he harm patients? I was very anxious my school would think the same about me.

The thing is, at our school there's not a middleman, a person who knows your side of the story and will mediate between you and your psychiatric care and the medical school administration. Some schools have this. The middlemen can turn to the admin people and say, "This person really can't take the test at this time." The medical school people, including the deans, should not have had to know the state of my depression, but they did.

Then after my third year I took a year off. During that year, they say that you still must be productive, so I did research at a hospital attached to a university. That was when I met a senior researcher in the microbiome department who is now one of my great mentors. He helped me see how awesome the PhD world is and I discovered that I really liked that style of learning.

It turned out that he had another project starting and he asked if I'd like to work on it. That led to me doing a PhD and I'm in my second year of that now.

But meanwhile, the year after leaving medical school, a pizzeria with a brewery attached was opening in town and I got to work there and I'm still doing that alongside my PhD. Everyone just pitched in and brought their suggestions to the table. I helped create the menu, form the ideas, and got to be part of that entrepreneurial spirit that I love. So now I know what it's like to open a restaurant!

I don't exactly know what I want to do yet, the restaurant business or research. It's an interesting question. But I'm realizing that MD-PhD is the right way to go. I enjoy thinking like a PhD and applying those skills to medicine.

For example, recently I went to an Individualized Medicine conference. It was cool to see all the genomic things that are happening, like computational research. But then you ask; "How can we get doctors to use these new research tools in the clinic?" I think I want to be some kind of intermediary between research and medicine.

So, I'll definitely finish my medical degree. My mentors there told me to do that because they say the fourth year is the easiest, and I still feel very attached to the medical school!

Some people think they'll forget what they learned if they have a break: I don't know. I was so depressed the whole time that nothing went in, so I didn't have that much to forget. I was at the fifth percentile! Now I am rebuilding. I took a ten-week summer course to learn medicine all over again and I enjoy it at this point. By the time I get back to residency, I want to be this bad ass, "I know my stuff" person.

I haven't quite figured out how everything will fit together. I have to work on myself right now. There are so many underlying issues that I grew up with that I didn't recognize as issues. It's just nice to take this time and learn how to be healthy. Being depressed and getting therapy is very different from like now, not being depressed and getting therapy!

Thinking back, there were multiple reasons for my depression. One of them was academically not performing as I needed to. That's hard for a student who has always succeeded. In undergrad, we were taught to study the concepts and not to bother with memorizing facts that you could just look up. I felt like I was going against my values in medical school by having to flat-out memorize things.

Then the social part was a problem too. I'd contact the girls on a Friday afternoon and they'd be like, "Oh man, we're just at the mall shopping." That was not me though. They identified me as someone that I didn't think I was. It took a while before I finally found my community.

Also, I think there's a whole cultural part where I was mad at my parents for pushing me into medicine. I should have been stronger and said, "No, I don't want to do medicine. I want to open this restaurant." Maybe if I had done the restaurant, I wouldn't have been failing. At the same time, I know that I now have a very enriched life. There are so many facets to consider!

My parents being of Chinese culture, they really don't get it. For example, a year after I stopped medical school, my mom said, "I don't understand. When you got depressed and had to take a break, why didn't you just go back to med school again?"

I was like, "Are you kidding me? There's no way I could have gone back to med school in that state." She has no insight about depression. A lot of people, if they're depressed, go home for a month to be with their parents in a safe environment. Not me though. I told my parents I wasn't going home, that I had some friends who would take care of me. Even now I'm working through my relationship with my parents.

My view of depression used to be of someone who can't get out of bed, who's not eating, or is overeating, or isn't brushing their teeth or can't take care of themselves. But really, that's not correct. Even a couple of weeks ago, I had a personal event that led to me having negative thoughts a lot of the time. Yet I still went to school, I was still taking my exams, I was still passing, getting good grades. You can still be depressed but be highly functioning.

But overall, I'm doing well, feeling pretty healthy and generally mentally stable. I've found a path that I like at grad school and even though I'm not ill, I always find things to talk about with my therapist, and I'm not ashamed about that—you learn a lot. I'll figure out the opening up a restaurant someday, or maybe that will always be just a pipedream, we'll see!

A lot of people don't get the mental help they need. I decided to tell my story because I've found it very helpful to know about other people in similar situations. Few people are willing to share their story of mental illness because of the stigma and potential consequences. I feel like it's much more open and more talked about in the PhD science world than in the MD environment. When I told people in grad school, it felt great that their response was like, "That was not weird at all," or "Oh, wait—that person went through something similar." So, it feels good and easy and comfortable talking about my experience right now!

**Discussion or Writing Prompts**

1 Describe how medicine is or is not a calling for you. What drives you to stick with it and get through difficult times? What has influenced your passion for your work over time?

2 Describe a time when you noticed someone who needed help, or when someone checked up on you.

3 "The medical school people, including the deans, should not have had to know the state of my depression, but they did." Discuss the tension between privacy and getting the appropriate support.

4 What is the value of self-discovery even if you are functioning and not depressed? How might a deeper understanding of oneself help navigate life as a healthcare professional?

5 Recall a time you had to navigate feeling that you didn't fit in or belong to a group. What helped?

6 Discuss vulnerability and sharing your vulnerabilities with others. What enables one to be brave enough to show vulnerability?

# 2  Anxiety

*Coping with anxiety attacks is an ongoing struggle for first-year medical student, Samantha Brody. But despite the challenges, Samantha is doing well in her studies and making friends. And with the help of counselors, she has learnt several tricks to deal with her anxiety that she wants to pass on to others.*

During the long road to medical school, I have struggled with anxiety. I had a very happy childhood, but sometimes anxious thoughts would pop up, especially as I became a teenager. Even in a very happy moment an anxious thought can come into my mind which I send on its way, but then it just comes back. [*Laugh*]

Going through junior year of college, I had extremely strenuous courses and I started getting anxiety attacks. They could be because of something stressful, or for no stress at all. My heart would start beating very fast and I would start breathing fast. Normally, it wasn't too extreme and unless somebody was really paying attention to me, they couldn't tell. The anxiety didn't affect my studies and I did well, but it was very hard to deal with.

The anxiety is continuing now in medical school. Sometimes, it happens in class, when there isn't anything stressful to provoke it, which is part of what makes it so frustrating. I think I have a really good perspective on school; I am focused on learning rather than grades. I consider my school performance important, but completely separate from my self-worth. I focus on collaborating with others and helping them also have fun learning, but I can still be feeling anxiety. I know that my body is responding inappropriately, so I have to deal with it.

When I'm having those anxious moments, I try to focus on my breathing and take a little mental break from whatever is going on around me. If I'm in a lecture, I stop paying attention to the lecture for 30 seconds. I focus on just taking a breath in, releasing a breath out, and acknowledging that I'm having anxious thoughts, or that my heart's racing, or that I'm breathing fast. I try not to get frustrated with myself.

At my undergrad school, we had free counseling and psychological services which were helpful and gave me some tools, like how to concentrate on

DOI: 10.4324/9781003475170-3

breathing. And I found it especially good to tell my friends and people close to me, so that if I was having an anxiety moment they could understand and be supportive. Here as well, counselling is free and confidential. But though I'm making friendships, I haven't quite reached the point where I'm comfortable talking about my anxiety, because I feel some people won't know how to deal with it.

When I'm having an anxiety attack and tell people, I don't want them to make me feel abnormal. Just take it as a matter of course, something that I struggle with but that doesn't define me. It is okay to ask me about it or ask what might be helpful to me. I might say, "I don't really need anything right now, but I just wanted to let you know." Someone else saying, "OK" and accepting me and then going on like nothing has changed is really important so I can feel like I'm not alone; that I'm not on the outside or different because of this.

Also, I have a life outside medical school. I've made it a priority to sleep because things are a lot worse when I don't sleep, but I do want to exercise more. I also make time to just not do much. Giving myself permission to say, "This is my break time; this is as important as the time I'm working," has been important for me.

I think there's a common attitude, even a culture, of taking pride in saying, "I didn't get much sleep because I was working all night." I think that's toxic for people who struggle with anxiety and also for everyone. Balance is the best way to learn and live while going through medical school.

If I met someone else who gets anxiety, I would definitely suggest they meet with a counselor or psychiatrist, especially if it's affecting other parts of their lives. There are some simple things that you can do with breathing and meditation, and there are also medications. The times I feel the worst are the times when no one else knows but me. Finding that trusted friend, that trusted group of friends or mentors is incredibly important.

And I would also say to people who struggle with depression, which currently I don't, but I have, that it's really tempting to think you're all alone, and that if you seek help, people will see you as less fit for what you want to do. But I've found that people are supportive when you tell them or when you seek help. Seeking help is often the most courageous thing you can do. For me, that's often the first step toward wellness.

I think my anxiety is going to make me a better doctor because I'm very empathetic when patients have anxiety, or when they show different emotions. I'm OK just sitting there and telling them, "I'm here with you." I know some parts of medicine tend to be more high speed and high stress than others, but I've been learning different ways to manage and minimize the stress and I think I'll be able to cope.

I wanted to talk about all this because it isn't discussed a lot. In my medical school, we had a session where we talked about stressors and physician depression and suicide and things like that but there weren't that many personal stories. I think it's important for people in the medical school class to know that the person sitting next to them could be depressed. The person sitting next to them could be struggling with anxiety. That person is me, and I am doing well! Or it could be you, and that's OK too!

---

**Discussion or Writing Prompts**

1 Explore your feelings toward people who suffer from an anxiety or depressive disorder. Do those feeling change depending on if it is yourself, your peer, or your patient? Explain.

2 Describe an interaction with a peer (or friend) with a mental health problem. How would you help them feel normal whilst encouraging help-seeking for their problems?

3 "The times I feel the worst are the times when no one else knows but me." Have you ever felt this way? How does someone know when they are safe to disclose a psychiatric disorder to peers or faculty? What are the risks of disclosure versus suffering in silence?

4 Samantha values her time away from studying and she prioritizes sleep. What are your strategies for coping with the stress of medical school?

# 3 Coping with Medical School Life

*Robin Smith is a third-year medical student. Despite the overwork and occasional dents to her confidence, she knows she is on the right career path. How she handles studying, dealing with colleagues and patients while maintaining a rich personal life offers a powerful insight into the medical student experience.*

Growing up, I watched my dad. He is a physician who loves his work, but also has balance in his life. Medicine was always on my mind back then. It seemed like something that I'd stumble into.

I was a chemistry major and as I started exploring other options, I realized I love to teach and considered being a chemistry teacher. I wasn't sure if I wanted to do medicine; it's a lot of school. Then I decided to be a nurse and I got my license as a certified nursing assistant one summer.

It made me realize that I might not be happy unless I did something in medicine, but I didn't know what. I did pre-reqs for nursing school and I started talking to physicians and realized that I found problem-solving and critical thinking very stimulating. I wanted to be the one putting the pieces together, so I decided, "OK. Even if I don't get into medical school, at least I want to try."

I took the MCAT once, didn't do great, and asked myself, "Is this really worth it? Should I redirect?" I felt like I should keep moving forward, but if at any point the door was clearly closed, I would reassess.

I retook my MCAT and did way better the second time. I applied to six medical schools thinking, "I'm probably not going to get in," but I ended up getting acceptances at two of them. Suddenly, I was going to medical school, and I had schools to choose from, which I never anticipated!

Every step and hurdle of the process helped me question if I was ready to really commit this much time, energy, and effort. And I kept getting back a "Yes!" Now it's an even more emphatic "YES." I feel like this is totally what I'm supposed to be doing! I'm in my third year of medical school and I'll graduate in about a year and a half, and then residency will depend on what specialty I go into.

DOI: 10.4324/9781003475170-4

There have been many difficulties. [*Laugh*] The first year of medical school, I was also planning my wedding, which was just a whole beast in itself! I didn't have the energy to really care about choosing flowers or tablecloths, so instead of concentrating on the day, I decided I would focus on developing my marriage and setting up our lives. Medical school takes a lot of adjusting to, and planning a wedding on top of that was almost too much. [*Laugh*]

Second-year medical school was a lot easier because the wedding was over, and I was living with my husband. I've learned how to cope and not have it seem life-ending if I do badly on something, or if I don't do as much studying as I'd planned. He is really good at pointing things out like, "You would've freaked out about this your first year, and now you say, 'Oh well, I did my best, gonna move on and do better the next time.'"

Each year of med school has been like starting over again, and with its own challenges. What you did in undergrad doesn't really count because it's totally different. First-year medical school, you have no clue what you're doing, but you're studying hard. Second year, you're stressing about taking Step 1 and how you balance that with studying for your normal coursework. Third year is absolutely nothing like the first two years, because you're supposed to show up and be competent and do whatever the residents tell you to do. But you don't even know what building you go to for your rotation. [*Laugh*] You don't know what to document when you write a SOAP note (method of documenting patient notes). You don't know how to do a good oral presentation. It's like starting medical school over again! What has really helped me is seeing whatever stage I'm in as just a season of life.

For me, one of the hardest things is studying. On days when my whole job is reading a book and taking notes, I feel super isolated and bummed. I'm energized by seeing patients and problem-solving, talking it through, seeing the clinical correlations, and understanding the academics behind it.

I think in third year, there are a lot of different challenges, but for me, the biggest adjustment is being comfortable with just not knowing everything, sometimes being made to look stupid and being OK with that, because it is all part of the learning process. I've grown to realize that the only way you learn medicine is by doing it and failing at it!

I think a huge shift for me was when I was on surgery and was hesitating to ask questions in the OR. I tried to be invisible because I was afraid of looking dumb in front of a bunch of people. Then I realized that this fear was making me miss out on learning and I decided I would rather look stupid and learn, than just get by and not feel stupid. You're a student; the answers won't always be obvious to you, so you must ask the questions.

Sometimes though, people can be intimidating. Just yesterday, I was in the OR with a robotic case; we could see the anatomy up on the screen. I asked, " Is this the uterine artery?" The resident was like, "Didn't you just take anatomy? Shouldn't you know this?" It wasn't that rude a comment, but it wasn't very supportive either!

In those moments, I've grown. Instead of being like, "I'm going to shut up because I don't want you to think I'm stupid," I was like, "Oh, yeah. We just took it but I'm trying to learn as much as I can from this case." People haven't been directly mean to me, but I've heard stories about that happening to classmates.

Another interesting adjustment has been learning how to be professional and not too emotionally invested, because I connect with people pretty quickly. When we were on the burns unit, this patient came in who had almost his total body surface area, 90%, burned after a car accident. We ran it like a normal trauma; did all the interventions we normally would. After all that, we pretty much decided that we could only offer him palliative care.

At that time, we didn't even know his name, and he passed away before we got in contact with his family. Because I thought it would be good learning, I went with the resident to deliver the news to the family. It was terrible.

It has been really sobering and humbling to realize we are in some of the most sacred and fragile moments of people's lives. I never want to become indifferent to that; I think that would be easy to happen. I'm trying to figure out how to maintain my professional distance, but also to be empathetic with patients and never let something that is life-changing or life-ruining for someone be just another symptom to me.

Like I just got off Gynecological Oncology. Those people give cancer diagnoses every day, but I'm on it for only a week. I'm like, "Oh my gosh. We're operating on this person because they had cervical cancer," or "This person has metastatic cancer and now has no brain function." My natural inclination, and the natural inclination of nearly every doctor, is to have a solution. But even if you cure a patient's cancer, that doesn't take away everything they have to walk through in the meantime, and how this affects them and their loved ones.

There are a couple of things I've learned to put all this in balance, but I know I'm naive. I'm a third-year medical student; I've been seeing patients for six months. I think that the best I can offer patients when things are hard is my presence, my hand to hold, or my listening ear. To say, "I'm probably not going to make it that much better, but I'll be with you. We'll take things as they come, and I'm going to fight this with you." I think that's therapeutic for me too, to just be OK with sometimes saying that I can't offer an answer. That's been my approach so far and hopefully it will play out well over life. I can't speak to how I'm going to handle it when I've been seeing patients for 20 years.

When I look at the big picture in medical school, it's really overwhelming. I keep reminding myself that we're pretty competent people and as things come along, you just make it work, one step at a time. It has been awesome for me in third year to realize that I'm capable of a lot more than I expected. Right now, I'm in OB/GYN so I need to show up on time and do my job, and I'll just take the next thing as it comes!

Long hours can be an issue, even though our school has limitations on the hours. I'm on GYN right now, and when I was on OB, we got there at 5:00 AM and probably left at 7:00 PM every day during the week, which was super great because you're caring for patients all day and literally delivering babies. But my job isn't just to show up and take care of patients. At the end of every rotation, we take a test. My job is also reading textbooks and doing practice questions and all these other things and finding that balance can be really tough. To every medical student and resident, I'd say, "Just be in the season you're in!"

When I was on transplant surgery, it was so hard. One week I worked 75 hours, and we had class for five hours, so 80 hours that week, and I was studying for my upcoming exam! But I reasoned that even if I got no sleep, it was only for four weeks. I got to hit the reset button at the end of those four weeks and readjust.

My husband has really helped me with that, because when life is crazy and I'm at the hospital for 75 hours, he can take on the grocery shopping and the cooking. When it's not that way, I can say, "Great, it's my turn to do them this week."

A huge thing for me now is realizing that medical school is the start of the rest of my life. This is my real life, happening right now! Life is not going to slow down and get easier. After residency, there's probably kids and even more work. If I don't take ownership of things, they're going to go away forever.

I'm training for a marathon right now: I run five days a week. If I'd just said, "I'm not going to run for 4 years because life is crazy," well, life is not going to lighten up and I'd never run again. [*Laugh*] My husband and I are in a small church group, and I could always have an excuse as to why I can't attend meetings because I'm too busy, but I make time. Medical school has really helped me hone what really matters and know to make those things a priority.

In undergrad, I got coffee with a different friend every day, but that's not realistic in medical school. So, who are my closest friends and how often can I realistically see them? I'm OK with knowing that that's what friendship looks like in medical school. Or I'll think, "OK, I need to get some sleep at night, so what can I cut out so I can actually rest and not be a grumpy, crazy person?" [*Laugh*] You need to be comfortable letting go of some things.

I wanted to talk about my experience because I think it's important for people in medicine to feel supported and hear another voice saying, "Me too." Everyone's journey in medicine is unique but the more we can understand and help each other out, the more beneficial it will be for us all. When you're in the weeds, studying or whatever, it's easy to forget why you're doing this. But the more I tell my story, the more certain I am that I'm headed in the right direction. In the midst of long hours or discouraging test results, it's good to be reminded why I'm on this path!

**Discussion or Writing Prompts**

1  Important events, such as marriage and children, will likely coincide with school, residency training, or career. Discuss the importance of thinking ahead and planning your path. How much is "life-planning" encouraged or quietly discouraged via the "hidden curriculum" in our learning environment?

2  "I've learned how to cope and not have it seem life-ending if I do badly on something, or if I don't do as much studying as I'd planned." Consider your experiences with perfectionism and coping with "good enough."

3  "What has really helped me is seeing whatever stage I'm in as just a season of life." Try framing the time in your life as a season of life. How can this approach be useful when thinking about your heavy workload?

4  "The resident was like, 'Didn't you just take anatomy? Shouldn't you know this?'" How would you feel if these questions were directed at you? As the resident, how might you have spoken to Robin? Explore the value of asking potentially "stupid" questions.

5  Describe examples where the power of a compassionate gesture was healing. How can medical professionals retain that skill?

6  "After residency, there's probably kids and even more work. If I don't take ownership of things, they're going to go away forever." How do you find ways to integrate your values or activities outside work into your day-to-day life?

7  What convinces you that medicine is the field you want to pursue? What gives meaning and joy to your journey?

# 4 A Medical School Dean's Perspective

*Dr Andrew Bart is a geriatrician and the dean of a large medical school. His memories of his own experiences have made him deeply empathetic to medical students' struggles.*

I was an engineer, so all my undergraduate experience involved solving difficult problems, getting credit for how you worked it out. It could be open book or open note—memorization certainly wasn't expected. Then I got a full-ride academic scholarship to medical school, so I thought, "OK, I can cope with medical school."

You get to medical school and find you're average, and that was fine with me; I was never competitive with others. I remember we had a practice anatomy exam, [*laugh*] I got a 34 percent! Whoa, I was not prepared for that! Each individual thing you learn is not challenging, but the sheer volume of information and the fact that you just must memorize and learn this foreign language of medicine was overwhelming.

We didn't have any resources, like tutors, to help us, at least not that was ever advertised. It was like, "Hey, we've given you a warning. You didn't do well on your practice exam, figure it out." I just said, "OK. I'll work harder, study differently, shut off my analytical brain and simply memorize." Then I did fine and got through the exam.

The first two years were really difficult and somewhat disheartening. Non-academic life was a bit empty. I had some good things; my religious community, my youth group, and a lot of long-distance telephone conversations with my future wife, which was a big support. But medical school was isolating, to say the least! There was an extremely competitive group that wanted to get honors in everything at the expense of others in the class. I kept them at arm's length. I had my own little group and we just wanted to pass the courses and get our physicians degree. It wasn't a cry for mediocrity, it was rather, "This pressure is insane."

It's funny, how my career came about. When I was a teenager, I went from thinking I would never be a doctor, to realizing I liked older people, especially after volunteering at the local VA long-term care facility. Then, at medical school, I found some amazing geriatricians who were wonderful mentors.

DOI: 10.4324/9781003475170-5

They really sustained me and made medical school great! One worked in a county hospital system with challenging, underserved patients and led the Elder Abuse and Neglect program for the entire city. I want to be like her one day!

Geriatricians are a special bunch. They do their internal medicine training, plus a specialty where they know they will make less money. They go into it for the love of the older person, almost uniformly. They have different drivers, not money nor prestige, and it's certainly not an easier option. It was really nice that I found my sub-tribe within medicine early on!

The more I learned about geriatrics, the more excited I got because it is both intellectually and socially challenging, with all the medical complications and social issues the patients face. I thought it was something I could see myself doing long term and that was correct; I still do it.

I also am certified in palliative care. When a 90-year-old or 100-year-old dies, giving somebody a good death, a good goodbye with their family, can be seen as a success; you get thank-you letters. I did ending-of-life care house calls for seven years and would get to know families very intimately with my old-fashioned doctor's black bag. About half of our patients would die each year and you certainly remember them with respect. Probably the most depressing experience of my training was not geriatrics, it was pediatrics, when you have children dying of cancer, or lives that get prematurely taken away.

There are aspects of my profession that still upset me. Why is geriatrics, that provides outstanding ending-of-life care, less well-regarded here than in some other countries? People say, "Why would you do that?" Even in residency, my mentors implied I was wasting my mind, "Why not become a cardiologist or gastroenterologist and make twice as much money?" I'd say, "I'm still making a six-figure salary. If that's not enough, then seven's not going to be."

I had some really upsetting experiences during my training, especially when I was a resident in the ICU. One of my ICU attending physicians created a horrific learning environment. He would yell and scream at people, and he was terrible at end-of-life care. We would do care that most people would consider futile, and he ran family meetings that were atrocious, where you'd be like, "I can't believe he just said that to a family." He wouldn't explain what was going on, wouldn't address the anxiety or the-elephant-in-the-room issues. You tried to patch things up later with the family when he wasn't around!

It was unthinkable to confront an attending physician in that era. You didn't say, "Stop yelling at me, your behavior is obnoxious." During those moments, you're just trying to get through the day. You knew you'd be off to the next rotation within a month, so the misery was time limited! [*Laugh*]

The ICU is not a very fun place when you're mad at the person who's supposed to be teaching you. We had one ICU attending who even used to steal our food! Opened the refrigerator, took food, it could be from someone's lunch, and just ate it during rounds with everyone watching! Just absurd behavior! You think, "I won't be like that when I grow up." [*Laugh*]

Now that I'm on the other side as a dean, I'm like, "Oh my god, I would fire that person!"

Camaraderie in your residency programs helps when a faculty member is a total ass, though we also teach our students to develop resilience, so they stay in control of their emotions if someone behaves badly. They need to let negativity flow out the other ear. If you're angry or crying because someone gave you a dressing down in public, you're not helpful to your patient. Instead, keep the patient in the center and see that light at the end of the tunnel. And take a vow, "No matter how tired I get, how exhausted I am, how annoyed I am with somebody, I'm never going to treat a trainee badly."

The time I came under the most tremendous stress and closest to burnout was when my mom passed away. She was young when she died of pulmonary fibrosis. She spent almost three months in the ICU on a lung transplant wait list. With my palliative care background, I led family conversations to ensure we all knew the game plan for when she got really sick, and that was helpful.

But even with all our training and experience, grieving is still grieving. Fortunately, I had great colleagues who were very supportive. But realizing how burned out I was feeling, I made the difficult decision to leave my job and move cities so my kids could be closer to their grandparents. That turned out great for my work-life balance!

Sometimes as physicians, we believe we are super-human. Doctors feel responsible for their students and patients and often come to work sick. I had a resident who once started an IV on themselves [*laugh*] because they had been vomiting with diarrhea. I was like, "You need to go home!"

I can't tell you the number of residents and students I have told, "Go home." A student once showed up to rotation when his mother had just died. He was in shock. We sent him home, got him support, and reassured him that his evaluation would not suffer.

Addressing work-life balance is crucial, as I've found out in my own career. Now we have all sorts of systems in place to help people. It's great to hear that our students are seeking out mental health professionals, counseling, and tutoring and are learning to recognize the early signs of burnout and fatigue. There is no shame or weakness in asking for help; it is a good thing that we encourage!

---

### Discussion or Writing Prompts

1  Dr Bart discovered he was "average" in medical school. Discuss your responses to similar situations.
2  "It wasn't a cry for mediocrity, it was rather, 'This pressure is insane.'" Explore the trade-offs needed with work in a high-pressure environment.

3 How important is salary when choosing your career?

4 Describe a role model who influenced your career.

5 Recall a time when someone your senior modeled what you thought was poor patient care. How did you deal with that? What would be helpful in that situation?

6 Describe a challenge with your learning environment. How are you learning to handle adversity or difficult scenarios?

7 Describe a time you were conflicted about making a change in your career or schedule due to stressful life events or illness. What helped you resolve the conflict?

8 Recall a difficult experience. Did you make time to process it with someone else, e.g., a peer, family member, or mental health professional? Why might you have hesitated to ask for help?

# Part II

# Culture of Medicine

# 5   The Brunt of Anger

*Dr Heather Lacey is nine years into her medical career, training to be a cardiologist. She hopes that her story will be helpful to others, who may be suffering in silence.*

When you're in training in medicine, there's this hierarchy and almost a hazing mentality or instances where you feel like you're the brunt of somebody else's anger.

I've noticed this throughout my career in different gradations and specialties. For instance, when I was in medical school, I remember being absolutely berated by a pediatric surgeon because of the way I interacted with a family member. I had never really been around kids before, so I was very awkward dealing with an infant as a patient.

Instead of giving me constructive criticism or help, he basically yelled at me in front of the parents and told me that I was no good in however many words. This was seven years ago but the feeling of being awkward and then yelled at is still with me.

And I can think of a handful of other times in my residency and fellowship training where someone above me in the hierarchy—usually an attending physician—behaved like this, coming down really hard and just yelling at me.

When I was younger in training, I thought it was a reflection on me. I'd failed somehow and deserved to be yelled at and needed to just suck it up and be better.

As I've gotten older and become more competent as a physician, I've come to realize that it wasn't a reflection of me. It was completely a reflection of that other person who was acting unprofessionally and inappropriately. That's changed how I respond to this sort of behavior. I remember when I was younger in training; you don't get enough sleep, you're overworked, and I'd frequently cry because of all the stress. Sometimes someone yelling at me would precipitate the tears.

I remember an instance in my fellowship last year when I was working with another service. This very senior physician used his clout to yell at me in the middle of the nurse's station in front of nurses and techs, reminding me of his stature in training.

DOI: 10.4324/9781003475170-7

My response as a fellow was so different than it was when I was a medical student and a resident. I sat listening to him yell thinking, "I'm not phased at all by this. He's making an ass of himself. He's trying to pin it on me."

I let him get it all out and I told him, "Thank you for sharing your concerns with me. In the future, we should probably do this in a private setting." I don't know how that would have gone over if I were a medical student, but as someone a little more seasoned, everything deescalated, and he apologized. Then we were able to go forward with patient care in a much more productive manner.

Yelling happens so often in medicine. It's not a reflection of the person being yelled at; it's totally a reflection of the other person. [*Laugh*] I think it just inflates them, makes them feel superior, like they're the better doctor. Nowadays, if yelling happens, I look for ways to deescalate the situation so as not to feel so bad and to get us back on track. Bad interpersonal behavior detracts from everyone's goal, which is to take care of the sick person.

But I can think of a few reasons why yelling happens in medical practice. It's a very high-pressure environment, so it's easy for people to get frustrated and lose their cool. It's very hierarchical, so if someone is tired and frustrated and something goes wrong, it's easy to yell at somebody under them. That person just has to sit there and take it; I think that's a set-up! Also, doctors are very prideful. They don't like to admit they've made a mistake or done something bad, or that something might be their fault, so I think there's a defensiveness, too.

So, you've got people who have an ego, who don't sleep very much, who work very, very hard and are very prideful, and don't like to admit when they're wrong. That all comes together when something is perceived as not going the way that they want it to go. Then they'll blame a trainee, or a colleague and yell at them.

As I evolve as a doctor, I try not to be the person who freaks out and I don't believe I've ever yelled at anyone. I try to never make anybody feel bad, whether it's the nursing or ancillary staff, other physicians, or trainees. I see medicine as a team sport and try very hard to be a good player and good communicator. I think that that's the most important, safest, and best way to practice medicine.

---

### Discussion or Writing Prompts

1 Describe a time at work or training where you felt like the brunt of someone's anger.
2 Think of ways you might respond to anger from a fellow healthcare professional. Does your response depend on how junior or senior you are?

3 "So, you've got people who have an ego, who don't sleep very much, who work very, very hard and are very prideful, and don't like to admit when they're wrong." Consider ways to productively respond to someone's anger by recognizing factors that led to it.

4 Think of examples of doctors being "prideful" and "defensive." Is there anything about the medical culture that either cultivates or diminishes defensiveness and pride?

5 Is it possible to reflect on your own mistakes and opportunities for improvement when someone is yelling at you? Describe a scenario in which you attempt to do that.

# 6 Competition, Balance and Happiness

*Dr Alan McKinney is a physician at the top of his profession, yet he clearly remembers back to the days when he was a young resident and life was made unnecessarily stressful by a highly competitive fellow trainee. Tragically, this man later took his own life. Dr McKinney reflects on the inherent pressures in medicine that can lead to such dreadful outcomes.*

I was a resident in a very competitive program with people who'd been all top of the class, several of whom had multiple degrees. And within the program itself there was competition. We would see patients as a group on rounds. We would go into a room and speak with the staff physician and questions would be asked about the patients we saw. Individual residents were responsible for specific patients, and we knew our own patients very well. But there was a co-resident who, to gain the edge, would read through charts and essentially try to answer questions about other residents' patients before the person responsible could do so. For example, the attending doc could say: "What did the MRI show," and the resident responsible would say something and then this other resident would chime in. Or he would correct the information that was given by the resident responsible for the patient.

Many of us within the program found that tremendously stressful. There was outright conflict because the people this individual would try to show up got quite disgusted and upset about his behavior. You're supposed to be a team working on something as opposed to an individual trying to move oneself forward.

One of the biggest issues was that this resident was "the chosen one," somebody who had gone to medical school at that same institution and was very much liked and well thought of by the senior people. So, though they had some discussion with him about the inappropriateness of what he was doing and the fact that it was leading to conflict with the other residents, we had to be careful.

As time went on, I and my co-residents became more confident in the things that we were doing, and his behavior became less of an issue. But

DOI: 10.4324/9781003475170-8

residency is a time where you want to feel togetherness; you're going through something that is unbearably stressful. Back then, there was no work-hour limit and we were working 36-hour shifts at times. We were taking call every third night, sometimes every second night, so camaraderie was really important. This person undermined that, but the rest of us got on tremendously and we've remained in touch over all these years.

All in medicine are high achievers, and you think that if you hit your milestones, you'll have success and happiness. But really it should be the journey that counts. Every step of the way, you think, "OK, I'm there." Then you realize, "Well, no. I'm not there." There is competition at every step. There is competition as residents, as junior faculty, as full faculty. No matter where you get to, you're going to be competing. The question is, how important is it for you to win or to beat the other person in the overall scheme of things? Everyone will answer that question differently.

But in the early years of training, I didn't see that. You try to make sense of why you are working so hard, up all night, and responsible for things that often you don't feel confident about. However, I think that's a crucial part of the journey. I think that the only way to develop confidence is to be required to make decisions under pressure. I can't say it was an enjoyable time. There was a tremendous stress on family, on personal time, on what is now called work-life balance, but I don't regret any aspect of it. I think that once you finish residency and start building your career, understanding that the journey is as important as the end result is really, really critical.

But here is the sad part of the story. The resident who was overly competitive died by suicide some years into his career. It was a tremendous shock for us. He was one of the most intelligent, high-achieving people I've ever met, and we saw no indications that he had an instability, nothing to suggest suicide at a later point in time. I wasn't in touch with him post-residency, but I heard about him occasionally. He had really accomplished a tremendous amount. I think that physicians have a much higher rate of suicide than many other professionals. A lot of that relates to the stress, anxiety, and the pressures we are under. Making mistakes in medicine is a lot different to making mistakes in many other fields: We must be held to a higher standard. How this individual dealt with that, why he took his own life, I just don't have an idea.

When I heard about the suicide, it was certainly a time for reflection. I reflected on how I deal with stress, how I deal with trying to achieve as much as I can and how I deal with the journey. When I've had my own problems, I've always had people to turn to. Hopefully, we all have those individuals. My wife is the first person I confide in, and I have good friends outside work who will listen. Also, I have multiple colleagues within my own profession, both inside and outside the institution and mentors that I'm very close to, so a great support network. But many doctors are afraid of being penalized in some way if they speak to the wrong person and I agree that you need to be careful who you confide in. That's part of the reason why having friends outside the institution becomes extremely important.

When I turned 48, I started reflecting carefully on what was important to me. The co-resident is not the only person I've known well who's passed away. I have many colleagues and friends who have passed away in their 50s, early 60s, a couple in their late 40s. As I got older, it became more and more apparent that you must really look at your life, what you're trying to achieve and where your happiness comes from. Does your happiness really come just from seeing patients or doing your research? Does your happiness come from your family and your kids? Does your happiness come from playing sports or doing some sort of hobby? Writing another paper was not necessarily going to be as critical to me as doing something for personal enjoyment. Success is not about achieving the end point; it's appreciating the journey. That took me many years to realize. I tell all my mentees and everybody I've trained, "Don't just go from point A to point B. Try to enjoy going from point A to point B."

---

### Discussion or Writing Prompts

1  Describe a time when the pursuit of a goal was a barrier to social connectedness or appreciation of the moment.

2  "I tell all my mentees and everybody I've trained, 'Don't just go from point A to point B. Try to enjoy going from point A to point B.'" What are the ways that someone can enjoy their work if it is highly stressful?

3  Consider a time that you felt isolated or didn't experience the camaraderie of your peers. Compare this to a time when you did feel supported.

4  Think about situations you have encountered when competition was unhealthy and worked to the detriment of the group. What could be done to improve things?

5  Where does your happiness come from? Are there barriers preventing or delaying you from achieving happiness? Can you see a way of overcoming the barriers?

6  Discuss Dr McKinney's statement, "I think that the only way to develop confidence is to be required to make decisions under pressure."

7  Think of a time when you felt anxious about sharing an issue with your work colleagues. What helps and hinders speaking up?

Would you feel less anxious talking with a trained peer support colleague? Do you have friends outside work that you can turn to for support?

8　Do you have suggestions for lowering the suicide incidence of physicians? What can/should the institution do to help? What can colleagues do to support a physician who they suspect is distressed or suicidal?

## Resource

American Foundation for Suicide Prevention. (n.d.). Support after suicide loss for healthcare professionals and organizations. https://afsp.org/support-after-suicide-loss-for-healthcare-professionals-and-organizations/

# 7   Suicide and Disenchantment

*When a close colleague took her own life, Andrea Johnson, a mid-career physician at a large teaching hospital was devasted, blaming herself for not recognizing the signs of her colleague's despair. But then it happened again. Another suicide by another physician. Now, Dr Johnson feels anger and disillusionment regarding a hospital system that, she believes, gives little support to doctors in trouble.*

I've been working at the hospital for 11 years and a recent experience has bothered me since it happened. It concerns a colleague that I socialized with outside work through common interests. My colleague randomly mentioned the idea of suicide with me and others multiple times in casual conversation, but I never thought it was serious.

Indeed, it happened. She died by suicide. If I had believed her comments were real, could I have prevented it or helped somehow?

As physicians, we know that if anybody mentions suicide, ideas of hurting oneself, it must be taken very seriously. With a colleague, another health professional, why did I not take it seriously? Why did I not do anything about it? I know of at least one other person who said, "How come we didn't believe those comments?" I just thought she didn't mean it because she used to joke and exaggerate. I didn't think she was asking for help.

I went through a period of guilt, feeling I should have done something. I wondered, what could I have done? Reached out to the Employee Hotline? Reached out to psychiatry specialists? I had to come to terms with realizing it was probably going to happen with or without my involvement and now I no longer feel guilty.

But I'm still thinking, if this happened again with another colleague, what can I do? If a physician is actively suicidal, that person could be confined to an institution and their career jeopardized. But career versus life.... I think I'm going to take life. At the hospital, there's an anonymous Support Hotline. If a co-worker says, "Hey, I'm going to kill myself," believe me, from now on, I'm ready to take down the information and call somebody. I'm going to assume that they're going to do it. I'm not going to take it lightly anymore. At least, I'm going to share the responsibility with somebody else.

DOI: 10.4324/9781003475170-9

Since then, another co-worker has died by suicide. He was not as close to me and never made such comments, that I know of. He was also somebody that seemed happy; he was the go-to person when somebody needed cheering up.

Suicide is just there at our fingertips. It happens at work, it happens to good families, to happy, healthy people. That's scary!

I don't think physicians are at a higher risk of feeling suicidal. I think physicians have easier ways, more access, or maybe are more decided to act on it. They are more likely to succeed because physicians are not going to cut their wrists. They know anatomy and if they're going to do it, they're going to do it right.

Life is stressful and so is the practice of medicine. We can't detach personal emotions from our professional interactions with patients. I think there has always been a stigma about being depressed, being sad, being burdened by emotions. Crying with a patient or crying with a family is a sign of weakness. When you realize, "Oh, I lost two or three patients today," you just must keep going. I suffer with every patient I lose, and I've been doing this for over ten years. I think there should be a way in the institution for physicians to grieve. How? I don't know. We provide lots of support to patients' families; I don't think we have that same support for physicians.

With the first suicide, the institution never talked about it. "Oh, it was an unexpected death," they said.

With the second suicide, the response from the department was, "A chaplain will be on-site if you want to reach out and talk." Really? That's just ridiculous! When are you going to find time to do that? Are you going to cancel your clinic patients to go talk to the chaplain? Make an appointment, wait in line? It's just not friendly or convenient.

Suicide is an illness. It's like having high blood pressure and taking medications. Somebody is suffering and decides to die by suicide. If they're successful, those of us that stay behind should talk about it in an open way, because if we don't acknowledge there's a problem, there's never going to be a solution. The more you try to hide it, the creepier it becomes, and the more people will speculate and try to find out what happened.

I think somebody—a psychiatrist, psychologist—should have talked to each of us who were close to those two individuals. Not make it optional, not make it after hours, not just tell us to call the 1-800 hotline. Somebody should have said, "You were friends or close with so and so. We need to talk to you; clear you to return to duty because you've gone through an emotional, stressful situation." Our appointments should have been cancelled to free up time for this. Not just, "Keep being productive in seeing patients and making money for the institution, and good luck dealing with this." The only person I spoke to about this was my spouse.

We are not just physicians, we're human beings. When terrible things happen, we become patients, and it shouldn't be up to us, the victims of the situation, to be proactive and have to decide if we need help or not. This should be a right and it should be provided.

I don't know how many staff have died by suicide in the history of this institution because nobody talks about it. Somebody must look at it. If the suicide rate is higher here than in other places, there's something seriously wrong. If nobody talks about it, we'll never know.

The way I call it is that I've fallen out of love with the institution. Initially I didn't see this as just a workplace; I saw it as my second home, my second family. The suicides alone didn't lead me to fall out of love. There have been changes in healthcare delivery, the costs, the rules and regulations, and the way this institution's practices operate. I don't know, maybe this had something to do with the two suicides.

In a way, maybe I should have seen this place for what it is, just a job, and that's where I am now. Regarding it as just a job, it's fine. When it's not fine, I'll find another one. I'm reorganizing my priorities.

---

### Discussion or Writing Prompts

1   What would you do if a colleague or classmate casually mentioned thoughts of suicide?
2   "If a physician is actively suicidal, that person could be confined to an institution and their career jeopardized." How true is this statement? Increasingly, mental health questions are being removed from licensure and credentialing applications. Discuss the ideal way for doctors to seek treatment without fear of jeopardizing their career. Include a real-life example, if applicable.
3   Describe your experiences of either having no space to process stressful clinical events and experiences, or times when you were encouraged to process emotions during the clinical day.
4   How do you expect leadership to respond after a colleague dies by suicide or another unexpected cause? What message is important to convey? What do you want to avoid?
5   Do you see your workplace/school as your second home/family or just a job? What are the advantages and disadvantages of viewing it as just a job? How does the way we practice clinical medicine today impact the culture and how we see our workplace?

---

## Resource

American Foundation for Suicide Prevention. (n.d.). Support after suicide loss for healthcare professionals and organizations. https://afsp.org/support-after-suicide-loss-for-healthcare-professionals-and-organizations/

# Part III

# Practice Challenges

# 8    Medication Error

*Dr Sara Ellis loves her work and is completing her specialist training. But a few years ago, she made a mistake with a medication dose that had the potential to hasten the death of a very sick patient. The incident left her traumatized for years. She's telling her story to help other trainees avoid a similar error and to help them deal with their emotions when things go wrong.*

This happened in my intern year—my first year ever working as a physician after medical school, and it took three years before I could even acknowledge it to somebody else because it was so, so emotional for me.

I was on the critical care unit, and we had a patient who was immunosuppressed from a transplant and came in with a very serious, multidrug-resistant bacterial blood infection. One that is very difficult to treat even if you are not immunosuppressed, so a very, very sick patient.

We were having issues with his blood pressure. He was on multiple medications, immunosuppressives, steroids to keep his blood pressure up, but we were still in trouble.

One day on rounds we were talking about his medications and the plan for the day. I suggested that maybe we should add stress dose steroids. I was very proud of myself because no one else had thought of this, and I was just the intern. Everyone thought this was a fantastic idea, so they said, "Go ahead. You can start stress dose steroids."

I put in the order. We were using an electronic health record, so when you type in the medication name it gives you different options for doses. I used that to help me guide the dose to give him.

There are two different kinds of steroids. There's hydrocortisone and Solu-Medrol. We usually do stress dose steroids with hydrocortisone. You can do it with Solu-Medrol, but it's a different dose.

I ordered Solu-Medrol, but I ordered it in a dose for hydrocortisone, which is basically an enormous dose of steroids. Nobody noticed this. The nurses didn't question the dose. The pharmacy didn't question it, even though it was not the correct dose for that medication.

DOI: 10.4324/9781003475170-11

The patient got this medication for two days. Then one of our nephrologists, a guru doctor there, sat down and said, "Who's trying to kill my patient? This is an enormous dose of steroids. Who did this?"

I remember my heart just sank, especially because he'd said, "Who's trying to kill my patient?" I realized that I'd made a huge error and it had gone through all the different checks and balances that medications are supposed to go through to catch errors like this, and it had gotten to the patient. It was a worst-case scenario. I very reluctantly said it was me. No one was mean to me about it, no one came down on me or anything, thank God, because I think I was hard enough on myself.

We stopped the steroids but he ultimately ended up passing away, presumably from this enormous load of infection that we never were able to clear. I don't think that my medication error contributed to his death, fortunately, but at that moment, I thought I killed the patient.

I briefly thought about telling the family, but I didn't go any further with that. I think, certainly, if it had been a larger player in what was going on, then it would have been necessary to tell them and the right thing to do. But in the grand scheme of things, it was one small issue in a very complex case.

I can't even describe in words right now the emotional toll that I felt. I went home and cried that night. I cried for weeks every time I thought about it. You always hear, "Don't let the interns kill anybody," and I didn't think that was ever a risk for me. In medical school and in residency they teach you the Swiss cheese model of errors where there's supposed to be all these checks and balances; and then an error happens that slides through all of them! I always thought, "That's not going to be me. Those huge medication errors, they've got to be so rare." I was one of the strongest interns in my class. I thought I was above those kinds of errors, but I wasn't. For at least a year, I thought I had killed somebody by that medication error.

I remember, after that, putting articles in my reading material about stress dose steroids. I put all kinds of resources in my phone about proper dosing. Even to this day, it's affected how I order medications. I'm never overly confident about doses; I always double check, even medicines that I use routinely. If I have any question, I always double check.

That first year, I got very emotional every time I thought about it. Only when some distance had passed could I go back and realize, "This guy was so, so sick coming in and, yeah, I made an error that was very bad and it got to the patient, but I don't think I have to carry the burden that I actively killed a person."

It was huge for me to go through that whole emotional process. I didn't tell any colleagues. I didn't tell my husband. I didn't tell any friends outside of medicine. I was so embarrassed. I was afraid to admit to anybody that I had done this because I felt very inadequate. I wanted to be a doctor, but maybe I couldn't cut it, maybe I shouldn't be doing the job, maybe I was dangerous? It was probably one of the most emotional things that had happened in my life, and I felt so guilty.

It took three years before I finally felt comfortable talking about this to other people. I was a senior resident by then, about to be in fellowship, and

I ended up sharing it with other interns. Interns make mistakes and I saw them getting emotional about it.

I found that talking about my mistake helped me to move past that error, and also helped junior people coming up who were worried about making errors themselves. I hoped that they would learn something from my story and be more cautious when putting in medication orders, realizing that they can't always depend on the pharmacy, the nurses, and all these other checkpoints to make sure that they're doing the right thing. We're all human and mistakes happen, but the most important thing is to acknowledge and learn from them so that you can move on and be a better doctor.

When my incident happened, the resident I was working with gave me some articles on stress dose steroids, so I'd know to give the correct dose in the future. But she never addressed that I must be feeling terrible about the error. After codes, we always are taught we should debrief, but there's never a formal process for it. I wonder if it would have been helpful to sit down with somebody and talk about it, but I also wonder if I was just so emotionally raw that I wouldn't have been ready to do that. I don't know if anything anyone said to me would have made me feel better.

However, it influenced how I deal with interns and people in training. When I was a resident and something bad happened to a patient, I'd do a mini debriefing. I say, "You're not the only one that something like this has happened to; there are people you can talk to." Not everyone wants to talk about things, but for that percentage that do, hopefully it would help them.

---

### Discussion or Writing Prompts

1  It is common for healthcare professionals to feel shame after a medical error. Describe a medical error you or someone else made and how you responded emotionally. What is the value of owning up to your mistake?

2  I remember my heart just sank, especially because he'd said, "Who's trying to kill my patient?" Describe how you would have handled the situation if you were the attending doctor who noticed a major medication error.

3  Dr Ellis went from thinking she would never make an error, to realizing that errors are always possible, even for excellent physicians. Explore your own experiences with humility versus being overly confident.

4  Discuss your experience with professional or peer support after stressful clinical events.

# 9    Commitment, Challenge and Control

*Dr Gary Redding is a senior physician approaching the end of a long, rewarding career working in several US towns in many specialties. He remembers 36-hour work-shifts and living in the "fishbowl" of a small community where he sensed he was getting exhausted and disillusioned. Then he realized that he needed to have three big 'C's' in his life: commitment, challenge and control. He's now a very happy man!*

I did my residency training many years ago, and back then we were placed on a specialty service for three months. There was no pyramid type system—everyone was equal. The other two residents were third-years, whereas I was in my first hospital rotation in nephrology. It was fairly complex work, and I was young, just 24.

I didn't understand what I was doing and I couldn't keep my thoughts coherent. I was becoming increasingly desperate and frustrated because this was the first time in my life that I felt incapable of doing something or had even questioned my ability to do it. Now I was facing failure.

If I had troubles, I could call the consultant at home, which was always a sign of weakness if you had to do that, but letting your patient die would be a bad thing too! Nowadays, there's always a third-year resident above you or some fellow around that you can talk to. At that time, there wasn't. There were no senior residents, just me. It was a tremendous responsibility.

There was a rule that any patient who'd had a kidney transplant and came to the emergency room must be seen by the duty nephrology resident, which was me. So, she came in, a patient with a fever and the emergency room called me to go down to talk to her. I examined her, ordered several tests, again still feeling completely overwhelmed.

Over the next two hours, as these tests came back and I began to organize my thinking, I realized that I actually did know what I was doing, that I understood the test results, that I knew what had happened to the woman; she had a urinary tract infection. So, I ultimately made the correct decisions, but that was because I found the ability to step back and look at the whole situation, to take a more holistic approach rather than just getting caught up in the

DOI: 10.4324/9781003475170-12

details. There was a *person* attached to it: She was very frightened about what was going on, she thought she was going to lose her kidney! She would have been terrified if she knew that I was three weeks into my residency, [*laugh*] but it worked out all right!

At that moment, I realized that I wasn't 'behind the eight ball,' I was ahead of it; I knew what was going on. Right then my whole attitude changed, and I developed confidence because I realized that this was something I was trained to do, and I had the capabilities. That experience has stayed with me the rest of my career. I've never had the feeling again of being totally lost, overwhelmed, and out of my league. If the despair I'd felt previously had stayed with me, it would have been awful. I would have really struggled and maybe thought about giving up, but I never questioned my career choice after that experience.

My first consultant for the rotation was a nephrologist and at the end of the three months I had him again and he commented that he was amazed at the progress I'd made; then it was evident that he'd been concerned about me at the beginning! Now he was impressed by how well I was doing and suggested that I take up nephrology as a subspecialty, which was a nice thing for him to say.

It made me realize how I really needed feedback at that point, someone to tell me I was doing OK. It's the Mid-West; we don't tell anybody how we really feel about things, but then this guy complimented me; it was incredibly encouraging!

Now as I teach residents and medical students, I make sure I give them feedback and praise when they're doing well. If there are things they need to change, it always must come with the message, "You're doing OK. Just look at this or that little part, but you're really doing OK." It's vitally important for them to hear this.

But I didn't take up nephrology. I did internal medicine rather than a subspecialty. Partly that was because of my obligations to a public health service scholarship that I got for two years in medical school. It meant that I had to stop my training at the end of what would be considered primary care, which for internal medicine is at three years. I had to leave the residency program and practice in a rural shortage area for a couple of years. By the time I was done with that, the thought of going back and doing a residency didn't interest me.

One of the jobs I got was in a small town in Illinois at a 200-bed hospital. I was in a 13-person group that had surgeons, family medicine people, gynecologists, pediatricians. I was the lone internist, which meant that every time someone really sick was admitted to the hospital, they were mine. I did all sorts of things that general internists could do at that time. I ran ventilators, put in central lines, did flexible sigmoidoscopies, as well as seeing patients.

It was the time when my wife and I had our first child, and I was doing everything good internists should do except sleep! I never slept through the night. I always had to go into the hospital at least once. Then after I came home, I would leave in the morning before my son got up and get home after he was in bed. And when I was on vacation, if I didn't leave town, everybody knew where I was. So basically, I would turn all the lights off, pull the shades, not answer the phone, and lie on the floor [*laugh*] because then people wouldn't know I was home! That was not a good way of managing my life. It was a small enough town that we were living in a "fishbowl"! Finally, I said, "I just can't do this anymore."

It's important to be able to set boundaries, to recognize that you only have a certain amount of energy to give to things, and you must save it for the right stuff. We need to look at ourselves honestly and say, "I can do this, I can't do that, and if I don't start saying 'No' to things, then I'm going to make myself sick." Financially, the town was not doing well and there really wasn't the possibility of adding a second internist, so I knew I had to leave. I found a different job in a different town, which turned out to be the institution where I am now working.

There are three traits that I see in many of my patients who are fatigued. They are people-pleasing perfectionists with a great sense of responsibility. They want to do everything correctly. They want to make things right if people are unhappy and they have this excessive sense of responsibility, so they need to do everything themselves. And those traits pretty much also describe everyone working in this hospital! That's why we went into medicine, but it's also the reason why we burn out. We don't have the ability to set boundaries.

There are three things that are predictive of burnout if they're not right, and they all start with C, so they are easy to remember: commitment to what you're doing; challenge, you have to be challenged and be able to rise to the occasion and feel that it's bringing out the best of you; control, you need to have some sense of this. Commitment, Challenge and Control! Thinking back to that first night with the kidney transplant patient when I had my epiphany moment, I realize that I was not in control at all. And though I was committed to what I was doing, I wasn't challenged; I was overwhelmed!

Since then, I've had three different careers within medicine to keep up my interest and to challenge myself. I've been a general internist and later became a Division Chair at this hospital. And now I've changed my career to something called "Integrative Medicine" that involves mind, body, and spirit. All these career changes have been to satisfy the three C's and everything's been great!

Telling my story feels very emotional because, even now, I see these big, powerful turning points in my life. It makes me realize that I've learned a lot from them. I think I'll just have to write a book someday because I have so many more stories to tell and share!

**Discussion and Writing Prompts**

1 "If I had troubles, I could call the consultant at home, which was always a sign of weakness if you had to do that." We now know that asking for help is a sign of strength rather than weakness, yet mastering something independently is also empowering and a critical developmental stage. Explore the tension between asking for help and struggling independently.

2 Describe a time you overcame self-doubt and felt competent. How does feeling competent reduce stress? How is competence different from perfection?

3 Describe a time when you benefitted from constructive feedback, or needed but didn't receive it.

4 What are your strategies for saying "No" and maintaining boundaries? How do you determine your approach to opportunities, requests, responsibilities, and the people you care about?

5 Dr Redding discovered that "people-pleasing perfectionists with a great sense of responsibility" are at risk for chronic fatigue. Discuss someone you know who fits this description.

6 How do you manage the feeling of being overwhelmed? How can you apply "Commitment, Challenge and Control" in your career currently?

7 Do you see value of incorporating an integrative approach involving mind, body and spirit? How could you implement this in your medical practice?

# 10 When Certainty Is Wrong

*As Dr Luis Ramos says, his "tale is worthy of a telenovela!" Now a distinguished neurologist, he recalls a story from medical school that he didn't dare discuss for a couple of decades due to the stigma surrounding neurological conditions.*

It was one of those very unusual circumstances and it hit me during training, something I would never have imagined in a million years! But it has basically guided my view of life ever since.

I was in medical school in New Orleans—and I wish I could make this stuff up. [*Laugh*] I was studying for a neuropathology final examination as a second-year and ended up having the exact symptoms of what I'm studying! Like I have this horrific headache. I take the test, and my next memory is waking up in an OR suite where there's a very nice nurse, who in my confusion and fog is saying, "Good morning, you just had this brain operation. You had this bleed and an AVM (arteriovenous malformation) and we took care of it all."

And I remember thinking, "Is this a cosmic joke?" It was just so bizarre! However, to make it even more interesting, the neurosurgeon who saw me in this urgent situation tells my wife and myself one of the worst things that you can tell anyone. He says, "You have a stage four glioblastoma, a brain tumor." But he hadn't gotten neuropathology results—that took another few days because of the weekend—but he was certain of it because of his experience. "It's the only thing it could be," he says. Well, I'm here 25 years later and he's dead. [*Laugh*] He was wrong!

The point is that story taught me two things. Number one; that things could have been vastly worse than having to spend a month in a hospital! Being given a mistaken diagnosis that it was the end of my life and then having that diagnosis completely overturned gives a lot of perspective on what's important and what's not. Number two; every time I find myself having to share something with patients, I'm harkened back to that experience. It has taught me how I would want to be treated, or my patients would want to be treated, in similar circumstances.

And that has been my guiding BC/AD story; before operation, after operation. It added perspective and informed my life and my practice.

DOI: 10.4324/9781003475170-13

Now, my wife would say it's the cause of all her mini-psychoanalysis therapy. [*Laugh*] I look at it more optimistically. She's actually a very good nurse and as I was in a state of semi-unconsciousness in the emergency room, she was convinced that something neurological was happening to me and tried to convince the emergency room physician of this. But he said she had to accept the fact that I was using illicit drugs, and that this was the consequence. I hadn't been using illicit drugs and I had no positive toxicology, but he reasoned that if you're a second-year medical student showing up with a headache and unconscious, it's because of illicit drugs and nothing else.

My wife obviously had a lot of anger, so after I'd had surgery and everything was corrected, she tracked that physician down in the emergency room. I'm like, "Well, I hope you shamed him," and she was like, "No, I just wanted to share, to make sure that he knows his diagnosis was wrong!"

So that experience has given us a special perspective, that in a weird way is an odd gift. I learnt several things from it. Number one, you must be open-minded about possibilities. Not everyone is going to have exactly what you think they have based on your experience. Number two, before you break bad news, do the most obvious thing in the world, make sure you have the facts. [*Laugh*] Never guess, don't take that chance because that moment is so powerful. I don't think physicians or health professionals realize that when people are in dependent positions, any piece of language, any gesture, takes on a magnitude that really is remembered for the rest of their lives. And number three, don't be patronizing. Just lay it out, be gentle, and put yourself in the patient's position.

What happened to me has actually done more good than harm over the long run because I'm like, "I'm studying neuropathology and I end up with a neurosurgical emergency; I have to take it as a sign from God to go into the neurosciences." [*Laugh*] Boy, was that an important guidepost! Luckily, I enjoyed doing it and I still love it!

Of course, it's extremely uncommon for a medical student to get the symptoms they're studying. I just won the wrong lottery. [*Laugh*] But hearing my story probably doesn't help their paranoia when it comes to wondering if they have what they're studying!

In medicine we are placed in a patient versus physician dichotomy; it's almost like you can never envision yourself as the patient. Often you assume that all the wonderful advice you're giving to patients doesn't apply to you. Before that whole thing happened to me, I didn't pay attention. But the truth is I had been having warning signs. I was having headaches, but I assumed I really needed to quit studying so late at night or something, but that had nothing to do with it! [*Laugh*] In retrospect, it was obvious, except to me! You have to be attuned to your body and pay attention.

I didn't tell people about the surgery for many, many years. I felt incredibly shy about it. [*Laugh*] People don't understand brain conditions or disorders and I think that the stigma surrounding them is alive and well, even now.

Maybe I'm mistaken in this, especially since I care for people who have these neurological conditions and I tell them to speak up about what they've got. But within the medical profession, because many professionals will connect it to a story that may or may not be pertinent to the individual, a neurological condition still has some aspect of stigma.

Also, if they're not in the field, medical professionals don't appreciate that a lot of neurological conditions are on spectrums ranging from perfectly functioning people to very debilitated people. And there are new therapies and understandings that perhaps have not been shared enough with the larger medical community. So physicians with neurological problems will hide them as long as they can and not seek medical attention. And that's even truer with our sister specialty psychiatry where, God forbid, if you show up and report depression, or some other type of psychological issue! It wasn't till recently that I've felt comfortable putting my own story out there, but now I find it oddly liberating and I'm glad I did!

---

### Discussion or Writing Prompts

1  Describe a time when being the patient gave you a different perspective on being a doctor.
2  What were the possible reasons that led to the doctor giving a premature and wrong diagnosis to the patient? Try to put yourself in that doctor's shoes.
3  Receiving a devastatingly incorrect diagnosis taught Dr Ramos, "how I would want to be treated, or my patients would want to be treated, in similar circumstances." What do you consider when reporting/discussing test results with a patient?
4  "In medicine we are placed in a patient versus physician dichotomy; it's almost like you can never envision yourself as the patient." Describe your feelings about being a patient or when you ignored symptoms.
5  Dr Ramos waited for many years before talking about his brain surgery due to perceived stigma. Describe your thoughts concerning stigma and illness. Is stigma a bigger problem for doctors than patients? When is it appropriate/not appropriate to share one's story?

# 11 Colleagues, Privacy and Empathy

*An unexpected stroke left Dr Graham Lawrence with functional impairment and his personal life in ruins. But returning to work as a rheumatologist in a major teaching hospital brought problems with his colleagues he hadn't anticipated. It also brought increased empathy and connection toward his patients.*

It was almost seven years back. I was in my 40s and I had a stroke out of the blue. No warning signs, no prior problems that would predispose me to it. It was an anatomical abnormality in my carotid artery, and it just tore open. All I remember is that people were bending over me; I didn't think there was anything wrong. Of course, I'm glad they didn't listen to me, and they called 911.

I argued with the ambulance guys to only take me to the hospital where I worked, and still work. I don't remember anything more. I woke up in the ICU a couple of days later as they were getting me off the ventilator, and then it was a long recovery. I got into the hospital in September, and I was there until late November. Then there was almost another year of outpatient recovery and physical therapy, and I got back to work a couple of years later.

It was an interesting experience in the hospital. When you are a patient in the place where you work, privacy is always a problem. Sometimes people are genuinely concerned, and they want to know what's happening, and some people are more like voyeurs. [*Uncomfortable laugh*] That is something that I became aware of.

One of my providers told me, "You should probably find out who has seen your medical records," because he mentioned that someone had asked him how I was doing and he had said, "Well, I can't really talk about it." Then he told me, "Maybe you should do an audit." So I asked medical records to do an audit and I found out that quite a few of my immediate colleagues had viewed my medical records around the day of the stroke or the next day. I didn't have any problem with that; I thought they were genuinely concerned. But when people were looking at my records two months afterward, I did feel bad. I didn't think there was any reason for them to be doing that then. I didn't want to make a big issue out of it, but still, if they wanted information, they could have come and asked me directly. They shouldn't have been prying, but I'm not surprised that it happened in a system like this.

DOI: 10.4324/9781003475170-14

But I felt bad. I'm a fairly private person; most of us are, so it made me angry. It would be natural for people in my situation to be angry, but I sublimated it. I informed the appropriate people and I think they probably told whoever looked at my records that they couldn't do it; I'm not sure what kind of disciplinary actions were taken against them.

Since I've returned to work, the problems with my colleagues have continued. Normally, people don't want to share what they have wrong with them but, in my case, the thing is so apparent; anyone can see that I'm partly disabled. You can't hide it and of course, everyone knows since I went through part of my recovery here.

Just to be fair to my colleagues, I understand that there would generally be a level of concern, and rightly so, as to whether I can work properly or not because of the neurological injury. But I think there are still a lot of psychological factors involved because physicians are always very anxious about seeing one of their colleagues get ill like that—it brings the issue of morbidity and mortality too close to home and that makes them very uncomfortable. I feel a lack of support here and though I don't want to use the word 'discrimination' because it is so inflammatory, I would say it probably accurately describes what is happening.

When I first came back to work, I had my neuropsychologist talk to my colleagues. And I don't know if any of the prejudice that is here now is partly because of that, because they know more about my cognitive deficits. I thought more information would actually help them be less prejudiced, but it was the opposite, which I found surprising. On the other hand, it's not as if ALL my colleagues are like that; the people who work in my immediate area are more critical, or more concerned, and the people who are farther away from my work area are much more supportive.

I've now been back at work a couple of years and my cognitive deficits don't affect my capacity to do my job. But you can't change other people's attitudes; the best you can do is to carry on working. I wanted to come back to take care of patients and that's what I really like. As long as my patients are happy with me…. if the patients start complaining, then I'll know it's time for me to stop working. But if there are no complaints, then it's fine. That's all I need to focus on. But I am lonely here in the hospital, without a doubt.

Since my stroke, the way I deal with my patients is very different, I think, to the way I behaved before. Now I empathize more and can understand the problems they face when they need to deal with the billing office and all the other annoyances. I am much more supportive, and I try to help them out if there is an issue like that.

What I have realized is that healthcare is so imperial. Trying to get a doctor's appointment is like trying to get an audience with the king. [*Laugh*] I think accessibility is something that we need to improve. I think if patients have more accessibility to their providers, they are more likely to be more compliant; it makes things much easier. So, I have made it a point to be more accessible. I have a separate cell phone line just for my patients that I give out, because half the time you're playing telephone tag; they call your office, they have to wait, they go through three or four different people, by the time the message gets to you, it's a day later and you get their voicemail, and then they go through the same thing again. So, I give them my cell phone number.

Patients do ask me, "What happened to you?" I tend not to get into my personal story with them too much, because obviously, they're not there to listen to me but to deal with their own problems, so I must constantly censor myself. Now I will share my story only if it is going to improve my therapeutic alliance with a particular patient.

But thinking about my own life, today I do a lot of meditation, more so than before my stroke. But I don't know if my own situation here will improve; only time will tell.

---

### Discussion or Writing Prompts

1 Describe a time when your privacy was invaded, you became aware of a boundary crossing with a patient, or when you were tempted to find out personal information about a colleague without directly asking them.

2 Dr Lawrence suspects that his colleagues were unsupportive because his condition triggered anxiety about their own morbidity and mortality. Think about a patient of yours who felt "too close to home." Examine your emotional reaction and how that affected your interactions with the person.

3 Consider a challenging personal experience that fostered empathy and kindness in your approach to your patients. How does that impact meaning and purpose at work?

4 What are the risks/benefits with providing patients with a dedicated cell phone number so they can reach you easily? How do you take care of your own needs and remain responsive to your patients' needs?

5 Describe a time when you shared personal information to benefit a patient and a time when you withheld personal information to benefit a patient.

6 Having an unexpected stroke catapulted Dr Lawrence into facing his mortality. What regret might you have if you were suddenly facing an early death? What changes might you make now to enhance meaning in your life?

# Part IV

# Career/Life Disruptions

# 12 Accident, Fear of Depression and a Great Career

*Dr Frances Horsham is a much-loved psychiatrist renowned for her generous spirit. As she nears the end of a long and rewarding career in private practice she reflects on her life, describing how she overcame depression.*

When I interviewed for medical school in Chicago, I was a French major; I didn't even have that much science. I had to go back for a year and a half to do chemistry, physics, and pre-medical and I said to the medical school dean, "I'm a French major. What are my chances?" He said, "Well, I was a history major." I thought, "That's it. I'm in!"

I was having a great time in my second year as a medical student. It was May 5th. I was riding my ten-speed bicycle, which I'd gotten the day before. I had trouble getting off the bike, but I'd listened to my boyfriend, who said, "You should get a male bike with that rod across it, one that comes up about an inch below your torso, so that you have the stability."

As it turns out, I had some books bound around the back with a bungee cord. It became unraveled and hooked in the rear wheels. I went flying off the bicycle and hit my right cheek, flexed it back, broke my neck, and was paralyzed from the neck down.

Ironically, I had worked in a rehabilitation center the summer before because I'd gone to see a doctor in rehab medicine about some scoliosis that I had. While he was examining me, a woman called and he said, "That's a very interesting woman."

I said, "How's that?" He said, "Well, she's a quadriplegic and she completely supports herself with a mouth-stick painting cards!" I was hooked, so I decided to do an externship in this rehab center after my first year of medical school.

I had talked to quadriplegics and paraplegics about the moment that they realized they were paralyzed. Nine months later, I'm lying on the ground, my teeth broken—I'm watching them go across the ground like Chiclets and blood spatter. I realize I can lift my neck, but I can't feel or move my legs.

So, I was taken to the hospital and gradually, over a period of about three years, I got back most of my mobility and most of my feeling. I was left with some residual spasticity in my right hand and a foot drop on my right leg. I was able to get my teeth replaced. I had a lid drop in the right eye that got

DOI: 10.4324/9781003475170-16

better. Gradually I improved, but I lost a year of medical school. And more significantly, I lost that sense of immortality and omnipotence that you have as a kid and a young adult when the world is your oyster. I suddenly realized that, in a split second, your whole life can be changed.

But the medical school and my teachers were incredibly supportive and my whole class showed up at the hospital. They were very humane, very committed to helping me get through!

And then the year after this happened, I had a whopper depression. This was because I had had my neck fused and I was doing a radiology rotation and wearing a really heavy smock to guard against the radiation. It ended up causing terrible spasms in my neck, spasms so bad that I felt like I was never going to be healthy. I didn't graduate with my class, which was a big loss that took a very long time to get over.

That big depression was very frightening because I just really felt hopeless. Finally, I felt so bad that I walked off a rotation in OB-GYN, and went straight to my dean's office and said, "I just have to take time off. I don't feel like myself." He said, "Wait. You're doing honors work." I said, "I may be doing honors work, but I've got to find me."

I left medical school not knowing if I was going to recover. I wanted to go back, but I just didn't know if it would happen. My injury and my depression were so bad that there was nothing more the school could have done, and they would have done more if they could have.

I went home to my parents and rehabbed. I got treatment and eventually returned to my life and survived all of it. It taught me a lot. I really worked on my hand to get the mobility back: I took guitar lessons and drawing lessons. I ended up getting better and better emotionally, and stronger and stronger physically. I just hung out until I was ready to go back to med school.

That experience influenced the direction of my career. I was always interested in psychiatry, but I was a little bit afraid of it because there's mental illness in my family. As a matter of fact, my mother died by suicide when I was 23. My brother had severe bipolar disorder, and he died in 2009 from the sequelae of the drugs that were used to treat his bipolar disorder.

I was afraid of having depression myself because I'd seen the ravages of it, but once I had had a depression and made it through, got treatment and went back to medical school, I wasn't afraid of psychiatry anymore. I've always enjoyed talking to people; I knew that was my forte and I have really had such a successful career afterward.

So, when I recovered from the depression, I felt like I'd been through so much that I could really understand what it's like to be on the other side of the bed or the other side of the couch. In fact, psychiatry had become very appealing to me. I loved all medicine. I loved doing surgery, I loved emergency medicine—ironic because it's so different to psychiatry—but mostly I loved talking to the patients. That was my favorite thing. Psychiatry just seemed like it was going to be right for me and it's been a great fit!

**Discussion or Writing Prompts**

1   Dr Horsham was a French major in college. Describe how applying the humanities or the arts benefitted your education or work as a healthcare professional.

2   Despite continuing to get good grades, a clinical depression forced Dr Horsham to take a year off. Recall a time you took, or should have taken, time away from work to reflect, rest, or recharge after a very stressful experience. How would you feel about sharing your story with others?

3   What personal experience helped inspire your chosen career path? Which aspect of your career is most fulfilling?

4   Reflect on the power of support from your peers or leadership. Include examples of seemingly small gestures that nonetheless show that they care.

# 13 Childhood in Foster Care

*Dr Joseph Binder is a resident physician who was raised in foster care because his parents had a substance use disorder. How he's coped with the losses and disruptions in his childhood and flourished into a level-headed young man is remarkable.*

I ended up in the foster care system largely due to extensive drug use by my parents and the shortcomings in their lives. They also inflicted physical and emotional abuse on one another, and my mother had mental illness. We were living in homeless shelters and on the street for several different periods in my childhood, and ultimately, it created an environment that was deemed too unsafe and unfavorable for me. After years of gradual decline in my mother's ability to care for me, I was placed in foster care, much to her reluctance. By then I was eight years old and she was my sole parent. My father was a lifelong criminal and absent most of my youth.

I recognized that I was a child and in no way capable of changing an adult's behavior, but I really tried to help my mother. The most compelling reason, I would have thought, for changing her behavior was our homelessness and the horrible circumstances she had placed us in. If that wasn't going to do it, then nothing I said was going to make a difference, but I tried. I vividly remember saying, "Hey, Mom, you don't have to do these drugs. You don't have to be with this abusive individual."

Her response was never one that satisfied me. She would often say, "These are adult matters," or "This is none of your business," that type of thing, so I knew that there was no changing her behavior.

I had a clearer understanding of my circumstances than children probably should have. I had experienced so much to that point that I was actually satisfied with the idea of being removed from the care of my mother and placed in a more stable situation.

Looking back, I can see that my attitude was very mature. I now have a newborn son of my own. I can't imagine him, years ahead, having a similar thought. I think it was bred out of circumstance and necessity, survival instinct, and things of that nature.

DOI: 10.4324/9781003475170-17

Fortunately, I was placed in a foster home with a relative who was very young, 26 years old. It was a great experience. It was a home where I could grow and feel like a child again, no longer assuming the role of an adult so prematurely. I could go about my normal pattern of development in a more typical way. I could identify with the idea of family or family unit for the first time, as mine had previously been so wildly disjointed.

Initially, I had a lot of anger related to my circumstance, and it took a certain amount of adjustment, particularly because I'm biracial —African American and Caucasian —and my foster family is Caucasian. I felt that it was sometimes a cultural struggle in identifying who I was and where I belonged in my family. But overall, it was a very good experience, and one that I'm very grateful for.

I decided to pursue medicine around my sophomore year in my home state college. I realized that I had overcome so much, and I wanted to make a tangible difference in the lives of other people. School wasn't challenging me enough and I felt that medicine was probably one of the most demanding fields that I could pursue and so I was led down that path. My choice certainly wasn't like that of a lot of my colleagues, who if you ask them, would probably say they decided in utero!

While my foster family was incredibly supportive, they hadn't achieved that level of education and I didn't have mentors at that time to provide me guidance, so I felt quite alone in pursuing such a high goal. I got into medical school and the next challenge I faced was leaving home to attend the school 1,700 miles away, far away from everything familiar. This was probably the most stressful and challenging circumstance of my life professionally and academically, even until now.

Quite early in the first year, I developed depression and horrible seasonal affective disorder. I had never experienced anything of that sort before. I think it was probably due to a multifactorial culmination of events; childhood trauma, rationalizing the idea of family and being then isolated from it, the move from a very warm part of the country to a very cold place that is socially very different, and the academic intensity of medical school. I was in such a disabled condition that I was unable to make friendships or personal connections, and I'm a very social person. I sought help quite early because I knew it was uncharacteristic for me to feel so bad. I reached out to family and to an incredible mentor I'd had a long time ago at college and he gave me tremendous guidance. All of that led to me taking one year away from medical school and returning home, and just re-evaluating if medicine was the path that I was still wanting to pursue, and it was!

I returned to medical school without any difficulties the following year. I was in better spirits and had new perspectives and was able to make incredible friendships that I still have today. Making friends was one of the keys to my positive change in feeling and behavior. I had pursued my goals at such a fast pace since my childhood that I'd never taken a moment to really reflect on all that had happened in my life. That year out was an incredible opportunity for me to compile my thoughts and energize myself so that I could be successful. That's exactly what I did.

I feared, early on, that there would be an attitude toward my depression, as though I were admitting weakness or inability to perform. That fear continued with me while I was on my break, and stayed until I returned to medical school and was successful. Then I found people I could speak to candidly and realized that talking about my former depression was exactly the right thing to do; it should be talked about more openly. I also realized that other people had experienced very similar things and that, while my institution was accepting, these sorts of issues often go undiscussed or not openly discussed.

Medical school and my career have gone very well so far, better than I could have ever imagined. I think there are a multitude of reasons for its success and an important one is the awareness I now have of myself. I'm comfortable and confident, and I know when to check in with myself and when to check in on others.

I'm now an internal medicine physician and I feel that I'm more well-rounded because of my self-awareness. I'll be practicing in primary care internal medicine for several years with the potential to go into a subspecialty soon. I think that I better understand the social determinants of healthcare because of my experiences.

I have a commitment to a nationwide organization, the National Health Service Corps, to provide care to the medically underserved. I have an opportunity to care for those in circumstances that I'm intimately familiar with, and I intend to give back to that community as best as I am able. No matter what field I end up in ultimately, I'll not forget my past experiences and I guarantee that they will impact both the type of care that I provide and my attitude to providing that care!

Meanwhile, I'm 28 years old and have lost contact with my mother, though I did in the past attempt to connect with her. She has never recovered from her illness and she has her own demons. It's not as emotionally taxing for me anymore, because I've spent more time outside her care than inside it. I have my own family now and my mother is not one that I care to bring into that situation. She belongs to a fairly dark part of my life that doesn't deserve continued acknowledgment.

I am proud of what I've achieved. The work is not done whatsoever, but I'm proud that I'm able to provide my son and my wife with a life that, as a child, I could have never imagined. For that reason, I'm very happy.

---

### Discussion or Writing Prompts

1  Think of a time that you chose a path or set a goal after overcoming hardship. What enabled you to conceive of, and achieve, your goal?
2  Despite extreme hardship in childhood, Dr Binder's first experience of debilitating depression was in medical school. Describe a time

when you experienced a low mood unexpectedly and why you did or didn't ask for help.

3 "I'd never taken a moment to really reflect on all that had happened in my life." Describe a time when you benefitted from pausing and reflecting on the feelings associated with a very stressful time.

4 Explore your feelings related to being isolated from your familiar, support networks.

5 Dr Binder ultimately realized he couldn't continue to try to fix his mother. Think about a time when your mood improved after you stopped trying to achieve an unattainable goal and focused your energy elsewhere.

6 Discuss how your past experiences shaped an aspect of the way you provide care to your patients.

# 14  From War-Torn Childhood to Life as a Foreign Medical Graduate

*Dr Basim Amin was born and raised in poverty in conflict-ridden Uganda, where slaughter and kidnapping were everyday realities. But education was his salvation and he worked hard to become a physician and then to go to the United States to further his medical experience. He has been in the United States for the past two years, training as a neurology resident at a large teaching hospital.*

My story begins in a small town in the northeastern part of Uganda called Soroti, where I was born. I'm the first child and my mom was aged 18 or 19 when she had me. She is a very strong pillar in my life but her relationship with my dad wasn't long lasting, mostly because of the war. At that time, the northeastern part of Uganda was heavy with rebel activity, so my dad had to move back to Kenya where he came from, leaving my mom. She did well to raise me and then later remarried to a soldier who knew that I was a very important part of her life, so he took very good care of us both.

We moved quite a lot because he was a front-liner in the army, and we were situated in a region with active fighting. He was an excellent gentleman. He already had two wives and children before my mom, which kind of complicated the situation a little, but he did a great job with me. My education though was very disjointed. Every time the rebel front was pushed back, we would move to the next town. When I reached the first year of high school, we had moved to a town called Gulu, really close to Sudan. I learned a lot throughout that time. I can fluently speak about six Ugandan languages because of that experience; it's helped me grow so much.

My high school was very good. It was built by Catholic missionaries, and it was the first time that I had been to a good school. But I was there at the time of heavy rebel activity. I vividly recall one night when the Kony rebels (the Lord's Resistance Army) came to take us from school. A few weeks prior to this, they had been to a girl's convent school in Aboke, where they stole 139 girls aged 13–16, and then they came to take us.

Fortunately, because of the experience of the Aboke girls, the government had put an army group in front of our school, and they fought back. We were in the middle of this huge fight that lasted all night. The army won so none of the students were taken, but then we had to be evacuated from school.

DOI: 10.4324/9781003475170-18

But, you know, a turning point in my life was when my stepdad got killed. [*Tearful*] I won't talk about the details of how he died, but our life had revolved around the military, the barracks, the housing, the support, even the school I attended. So, then my mom had to take us back to where she came from. At that point, she had three more children and we returned to my birthplace to reside with her parents. In Africa, if a girl gets divorced or loses a husband, the practice is to go back to your dad's home, so that's what she did. But he didn't have much himself; he had a small place and we all camped there together. Two of my mom's sisters were also at home with their children. So, we had this huge family all growing up together.

It was good in a way, but it was very tough, very different from what we were accustomed to. It was really hard because my mom has absolutely zero education, but she had to fend for us children. I'm very proud of her! [*Emotional*]

When my stepdad died, I spent a year out of school, but my mom worked hard to pay for our education and fast forward, I was admitted to study sciences in a senior high school. Our education system is modeled on the British system and when you finished high school and applied to university, you were allowed four choices of what you wanted to study. I wanted to teach high school science because growing up, my teachers were my mentors and I looked up to them. But when I took my forms to the school office, my career guidance teacher said, "No, you shouldn't put education first and nursing second. You have the ability to score well enough to get into medicine." I hadn't considered medicine, not because I didn't want to do it, but mainly because I didn't think I'd get into it.

Long story short, when the results came out, I was pleasantly surprised to be accepted to study medicine in Mbarara with sponsorship from the government. And that's when things changed for me. So that's how I ended up as a doctor, because of that one teacher who had me change my university choice.

When you finish medical school, you can choose where you want to do your internship. I requested to be posted back to my hometown, so I went back to Soroti and it was the most fulfilling year of my life. I was being trained, I was treating my own people, and my family had such pride!

Then I was fortunate enough to get a job at the teaching hospital back in Mbarara. So I returned to my medical school on the other side of the country and taught there for one year and I was enrolled for residency. I did three years of residency in internal medicine, and I was retained by the university to continue teaching. I felt that that was the ultimate peak of my achievements. I was like, "Yay. I'm teaching. I'm a doctor." In Uganda, neurology is part of internal medicine, and I was working on the neurology ward in 2015 when I met physicians from the US who go there once a year to teach clinical research and clinical care. I expressed interest in getting additional training in neurology and the lady said, "Oh yeah, you can do that in the US and I can probably help you, but you'll have to pass XYZ exams first."

I didn't know much about the US exam requirements, so I looked them up and I also looked for alternative routes to get neurology training and there was nothing else. There are some training programs in South Africa, North Africa, Egypt, and the like, but none in East Africa. In my country there were only two neurologists for 40 million people, one of whom was my mentor. He was a British neurologist who'd retired from London to work in Uganda a decade or more before. I worked closely with him and felt that I wanted to do this type of work enough to go through the pain of sitting the exams that get you into a US residency position. So, I prepared for and sat the exams — steps one, two, and three of the United States Medical Licensing Examination and I passed them!

And that's how I got here. I was invited to interview at three places, and I picked here mainly because of the relationship that I had built with the team that went over to Mbarara all those years ago. I think, honestly, if you told me ten years ago that I would be in the United States, I would have called you crazy!

The first few months here were rough. I came from a health care system in Africa where there were no electronic health records, and in the United States I had to do everything on the computer; put in orders, write notes. I would come in very early and stay up until late. Also, I had to adapt to the language, which sounds different from the English spoken in my country. I was having to learn to communicate with patients and my peers so they wouldn't need to listen and then say, "Could you repeat it?" And I found it difficult to follow conversations. I remember calling one of my friends and saying, "I thought I knew English, but I don't. People talk fast and I'm having to repeat myself all the time."

Now that I've been here for two years, I think it's been an excellent learning opportunity and experience. The facilities are world class, the patients are great. The teachers are very competent, willing to help, and we have a program director who is always available. I have a strong support system here. The team that visited Uganda works at my institution and they've continued to mentor and stay close to me, both in medicine and outside of medicine. But then, just when I started to feel that this is nice, it feels like home, the racial tensions started to peak in this country. That was rough to take in and it still feels uncomfortable.

Luckily, I haven't directly experienced racism. Perhaps micro things but nothing direct, thankfully, but I feel worried. I'm afraid of cops because of some well-publicized incidents in different states. I try to make sure that my car has everything it needs, and I just try to avoid interacting with a cop. I have a wife and two children and when we are at home, I fear that the police could break into the house and harm us because of mistaken identity. So, I don't feel safe on the road, and I don't feel safe in our own house.

I don't know if I will stay in the United States. My goal is to go back home and contribute to my country and be with my mother. When that will be will depend on circumstances. Now I have two more years left and then I'll do two more years after the fellowship, most likely here as well. It would have to be the right job for me to move back home, so I might stay here for a while. But not indefinitely because I don't think that this is a place where I can be comfortable forever.

My wife was a doctor back home. She's my best companion and very supportive. She was at the very top of public health in Uganda, making decisions for the entire country regarding where HIV money should be spent and things like that. She was earning probably three times the amount of money I was making when I was working at a public institution. So, she left all that to come here with me and stay at home. But fortunately, once we got here, she went back to school and did a masters in the science of healthcare delivery. She finished in May this year and her goal in life is to do a PhD in global health work and then contribute to the public health challenges of East Africa. Currently, though she's doing research. She's got contacts and she's happy, so that's fantastic! But like me, she cannot wait to get back home, to take our kids to see their relatives and spend time with the family. We are starting to belong to both countries, so this gives us interesting choices.

---

**Discussion or Writing Prompts**

1 We often do not know much about a colleague's past personal experiences. Discuss a time you felt closer to a colleague or friend after finding out about their life or past.

2 Even though Dr Amin's mother had little education, she was a strong inspiration and he felt proud of her. Who was an inspiring role model in your life? Why?

3 Recall when someone saw potential in you; or conversely, how you have encouraged another person to see potential in themselves.

4 Dr Amin created an opportunity to enhance his career after meeting physicians from the US who were in Uganda to teach in his program. The cognitive scientist, Maya Shankar, describes 'imaginative courage' as being unafraid to ask the questions that open up opportunities. Describe a time when you had 'imaginative courage.'

5 "I just try to avoid interacting with a cop... I fear that the police could break into the house and harm us because of mistaken identity." Discuss the impact of constant stress associated with fear of being targeted due to race, gender, or other identifiers. What are some ways to guard against unfairly pre-judging someone?

6 How do you feel about moving far from home to enhance your career? What personal qualities or external conditions are helpful when making such a transition? What makes your career path a calling and how much might you be willing to endure for it?

7 Describe your experience with the trade-offs in a dual professional relationship and how you addressed each other's needs.

# 15 Empathizing with Mentally Ill People

*Dr Tara Woodstock is a mid-career internist, deeply embedded in her local community. She cried as she spoke about her brother's schizophrenia and how that makes her empathize with patients coping with mental illness.*

My brother has mental health issues that didn't come out until I was in residency. He is now in his 30s, living with my parents and is considered seriously mentally ill. He won't ever be a functioning member of society. He probably is schizophrenic, but part of his personality disorder is that it's hard for him to recognize his problems. He has a lot of issues with psychiatrists and physicians, so he hasn't had a formal diagnosis.

My brother was homeless for a significant period, living on the street. Because of him, I know how important it is to look after mentally ill people. It has been beautiful for me to be able to go into the city and take care of homeless patients there. I'm so grateful to the professionals and volunteers who do that work regularly.

Seeing my brother's experience affects how I approach my colleagues and patients who have mental health problems. As physicians, we push through a lot and work hard and have high expectations. It's good to recognize that we are human, and how dealing with mental health issues can set you back just like they do anybody else. Being able to take those experiences and empathize with people is so valuable. The patients may not have had the same experiences, but understanding how difficult circumstances can impact their lives certainly makes me a better doctor.

Sometimes I get upset and emotional when I hear stories that remind me of my brother's life, though I have gotten better about it over time. How do you translate your feelings from sadness or sorrow to empathy with your patients without showing too much emotion? As a physician, I think it's important to be empathetic, but I don't want to be too devastated. I must be there for my patients, not have them feel like they need to take care of me at some point. I try my best not to expose this side of me, because it looks weak.

Ironically, I tell my patients that feeling upset has nothing to do with how strong you are, it is because something impacts you deeply, but as a physician, I can't let my feelings show. I should save my emotions for scenarios like [*laughs*] this story!

DOI: 10.4324/9781003475170-19

**Discussion or Writing Prompts**

1   How has a family member's or friend's illness influenced your approach to your career, colleagues, and patients?
2   Describe situations where you contained strong emotions evoked by your patient's story. Does suppression of emotions impact your ability to be empathetic?
3   "…as a physician, I can't let my feelings show. I should save my emotions for scenarios like [*laugh*] this story!" Where do you find appropriate places to show emotions aroused by your work with patients?
4   Explain how you feel about caring for vulnerable or marginalized people. How did you develop your attitudes?

# Part V

# Women in Medicine

# 16 Infertile and Fulfilled

*Dr Ann Sunshine shares how she had to confront the pain of childlessness. Now she advises other women physicians to be aware of their declining fertility as they concentrate on developing their careers. She also mentors women juggling home responsibilities and their professional lives in medicine.*

I always wanted children, in fact, I wanted three. I had had it in my mind forever because I come from a family of three. But I delayed having children after I got married so I could complete school. Then when I was 34, everything seemed right and I got pregnant very quickly, but I had a miscarriage at ten weeks.

It turned out that the marriage wasn't good, and after my miscarriage I really didn't want to bring a child into it, and we ended up getting divorced when I was 36. Then I was a woman on a mission. I asked everybody I dated, "Do you want children?" I interviewed them, basically!

I was really gun-shy about getting married again, but I didn't meet anybody that I felt was appropriate. So, I tried to get pregnant on my own, starting when I was 40. I certainly had misgivings about having a baby on my own, but even so, I tried. I used artificial insemination a few times, but it didn't work.

So then, I went out with several people, all of whom, for some reason, wanted to give me a baby. Two men I went out with even had their vasectomies reversed! [*Laugh*] It used to be a joke—don't go out with her because you're going to have to go under the knife again! [*Laugh*] Thank heaven, I didn't get pregnant—it would have been a bad deal having a baby with those people!

The years just passed, and it was devastating. It was the hardest thing because I really felt like, "How can I live without a child?" Some people don't care about having children, but I certainly did. But I didn't want to adopt; I just didn't want to do that.

When I was 44 years old, I went with a girlfriend to Disneyland. She wanted to go—it was like putting me in hell! But it turned out to be good because it was the final catharsis that I wasn't going to have a child of my own.

I just got back from that trip and got a call from the daughter of one of my good friends who said, "I'm pregnant." She was only 18 and not married. She said,

DOI: 10.4324/9781003475170-21

"I know you can't have children," which was the first time somebody had said that to me. She said, "But you have so much to offer a child that I would love for you to be the godmother to my baby and have a real impact in his or her life."

That was the first child that I was a godmother to. Then my secretary's daughter had a baby, and I was the godmother. Then there was a young woman whose father I dated when she was 15. Her parents were divorced, and she went to live with him. Her mother was a severe alcoholic, very abusive.

Her father and I only dated for six months, but this young woman really needed a female role model, and I became like a big sister to her. Eventually, Anna just called me "Mom" and she became like my daughter. She's a teacher now and lived with me a few years ago. She's like a fantastic, real daughter!

Then I married for the second time and my new husband had a teenage son called Luke. When I came into the picture, Luke didn't have a relationship with his mother; he was a lost kid who really needed a mom. We developed a very close relationship and I realized he had some problems with alcohol and drugs. We got him into treatment—that was 13-and-a-half years ago. He has not had one slip since then and Luke is truly my kid!

And since then, it's like kids came out of the woodwork. Children of friends who now call us Grandma and Grandpa. When I was asked to help lead a support group for physician moms at the hospital I said to my colleague, "But I haven't had my own children," and she said, "Ann, you're a mom; you are like one of the biggest moms I know!" And that has been so great because I have all these young women physicians and PA's that I get to mentor and pass on all this advice.

What I tell young women now is; "Have your babies because there's a drop in fertility at 34, and there's another profound drop at 37," which I didn't realize even though I'm a doctor. I got pregnant at 34, but by 40 when I started trying again, it was already late. Possibly, if I'd done IVF I might have had a baby, but it's so expensive and I was alone at that point, between marriages. I think it's important to have your children when you're younger.

But women in the medical field often delay having children. Women in medicine and in the professions get this delusion that they can do anything because they've had successes like getting good grades and getting into medical school. There's a lot of power in being a physician—you call the shots—but you can't screw with Mother Nature!

One of the things I did while working at this hospital was to start the *Resident Stress Committee*. I would get a call, usually in November, after the new interns and residents had started in July. Somebody would be having a breakdown. And a lot of why they were having one was because of all the stress of moving here from elsewhere. They maybe had small children at home, and resident schedules used to be brutal.

Now I have a young woman who's an intern and she's doing a family practice residency. She has a new baby, about six months old, and his sleep got completely disrupted when she moved here. She's still breastfeeding, and it's just been ridiculously difficult for her. Fortunately, her program is very humane so she can pump whenever she needs to, and they try to give her a better schedule. But there needs to be an understanding that it's not just for a woman's family that she is taking some time off or having changed schedules. It also benefits work and society.

Often the women come to my group meeting and say that they are only working 80%. But if they had a different job, not in medicine, the hours they're doing would be much more than full time! I think we need more awareness of the extra responsibilities these women face. The suicide rate among women physicians is up to 240% higher than in the general population. Among male physicians, it's up to 80% higher depending on the study. In this hospital we lost two doctors last year. Part of the reason is the shame they feel because they don't want to admit that they're at breaking point. Part of it is chemical dependency; there's a higher rate of chemical dependency among physicians because drugs are available. Also, it's all the stress, the drinking, and the workaholism.

So, I think physicians and students need to be educated about this, because there's so much shame in not being perfect and not being able to do it all. And of course, it's a myth that you can do it all! It ultimately falls upon a woman to do a lot of the caretaking; planning the dinners, preparing the snacks for the kids, making sure they get to their medical appointments, and such stuff. I don't think men see the same needs that women see. If you're a woman physician, you want to give fantastic care to your patients, but then you must go home and do the whole thing there too!

I think that there needs to be education beginning in medical school about what life is like as a physician. Young people entering the profession don't know that there can be many challenges as well as all the rewards. Telling this story has made me think more about my life and the lives of other physicians, especially working women. I've come to terms with my own life and I'm very happy now. My mantra when I was 41 used to be, "I'm 41, barren and alone." My mantra, I think, now would be, "I'm 69, abundant, and surrounded with love!"

---

### Discussion or Writing Prompts

1 Consider the benefits of delaying pregnancy to get through medical school and training versus increased risk of infertility. How much of that decision is personal versus lack of support in the culture of medicine?

2 "But women in the medical field often delay having children." How important is fertility planning? Do schools and residency training programs adequately support pregnancy and raising a child during training? What does your institution offer? What is the ideal scenario?

3   Does having children when in school or training impact men and women differently? If so, how?

4   What are the pros and cons of reducing FTE (full-time equivalent) for managing family life? Are there other options? Does your response vary depending on the gender of the physician? Explain.

5   Discuss Dr Sunshine's statement, "…there's so much shame in not being perfect and not being able to do it all."

6   What enabled Dr Sunshine to evolve from "I'm 41, barren and alone" to "I'm 69, abundant, and surrounded with love!"?

# 17  Finding Balance with Kids and Career

*A demanding career, bringing up children, and maintaining a marriage was quite a challenge for radiation oncologist, Dr Jessica Haverford. She's always been very successful in her work, but that carried a cost for her personal life. She eventually came through, stronger and happier than ever.*

My day job is as a radiation oncologist, but I've had many different administrative and leadership roles the whole time. That led to a lot of job fulfillment since I've always had something else as an outlet for my passions, in addition to taking care of patients. It's kept me from being burned out because there's a high rate of burnout in radiation oncology. But it also creates tensions because sometimes you get over-committed and then you get stressed out. You need to step back and try to rebalance. One of the biggest stressors is trying to cope with work alongside marriage and motherhood.

I have three children who are all out of the house now. They're 25, 23, and 21. It's exhausting when you have three kids, each two years apart, but on the other hand, it does regenerate you and it gave me strength and joy. When they were little, I was balancing a busy clinical practice with my very substantial administrative roles that required a lot of travel, and having a husband who was in medicine and working in the same place as me. It didn't leave time for much else, not even for exercise.

There's a lot of guilt with trying to juggle work and motherhood. All mothers feel this. There were times when I would miss school parties and the after-school performances. I remember traveling on my two-year-old's birthday, and I felt terrible. I beat myself up! Now that he's 25, I can say he would have no clue that I wasn't there. [*Laugh*]

It's really fatiguing when you're trying to be the best that you can be at home and also the best you can be at work. And it's challenging when you're trying to have a marriage on top of that. I actually wound up getting divorced from a husband who decided that he wanted to move on and find someone younger and different. And this was when my children were in middle school and grade school. It was one of my biggest life-blows.

There were several factors that led to the divorce. When you are both really busy, you can get in your own orbits and maybe lose connectivity.

DOI: 10.4324/9781003475170-22

Then sometimes, when you have kids, all the focus goes on them, and you can lose the pair connectivity too. Also, it can be a bit difficult if the woman in the relationship has more accolades or leadership opportunities than the male. Some men in the partnership find that challenging. Mine did.

When you have a major a blow like a marriage going wrong, it's sometimes hard to bounce back. You have to give yourself permission to take time off and breathe, and then just inwardly focus and re-evaluate what's important in your life.

One of the things that helps during those stressful periods is having friends at work you can talk to. If you are not feeling quite all-that-together one day, they'll have your back. Also, having friends outside work is important so that medicine isn't your entire world and there are people around you that have other interests, that disconnect you from your day-to-day business.

Another lesson that I've learned is that many times, stressors in your career in medicine can come from insecurities. I started off fairly young doing my administrative duties, and I knew that most people had more experience than me. I remember just endlessly evaluating, "Oh, I shouldn't have said that in a meeting," or "I should have presented differently," or "You seem too nervous. You seem insecure of your...." You mentally beat yourself up. People on the outside don't necessarily see it, but you have this inner voice that keeps tearing you down about what you should have done differently.

Once you get a bit older, you stop worrying so much about what other people think of you. You just say to yourself, "Well, that's it. That's the way I am and here I go." That can remove some of the stress.

Also, comparing yourself to other people when you're early in your career can be painful, particularly when you're in academic medicine. Other people may be publishing more or presenting more, have more of a national reputation. You think, "Why can't I do that?" After a while, you either figure, "I can do it too," and do it, or you decide it's really not important. Sometimes finding what's important takes a while. I would just say, be kind and compassionate to yourself.

In medicine, there's sometimes what I call a "boot-camp mentality," where it's like, "Well, I've done it, and you should do it too." In my department, it wasn't really like that. Sometimes I would just tell my chair, "I've got to go. I've got a volleyball game for my kid." They're like, "Yeah, that's fine as long as you get your work done." Sometimes if you just ask to leave early or have the day off you can find that flexibility.

You find ways of balancing, but sometimes, it requires creativity to do what you want to do! I'm now happily remarried, and my current husband always laughs at me because I was famous for finishing my last patient, running out, changing in the car as I'm driving. At a stop light, I'd pull off my pantyhose and skirt and put on a pair of shorts or pants to go to a volleyball game. He was like, "I'm not going to bail you out when you get arrested for indecent exposure." [*Laugh*]

I chose radiation oncology because I knew I wanted to have a family. I got to the end of my junior year in medical school, and I didn't like anything that I had gone through, not the content nor the lifestyle. I thought, "Well, you're in trouble." I kept going until I found a specialty that gave me regular hours of patient care time and that didn't take me out a lot at night. Luckily, I've loved my specialty.

But giving bad news is a strain. Over time, you get better at doing it. It's not that you get calloused toward giving bad news; it's just that after a while, you find a way of insulating yourself. The key is to be empathetic toward people and show warmth and caring, but at the same time, you try to build up a wall in your own heart so that it doesn't take you down.

The hardest time is when you're treating friends. I had a very close friend who was about ten years younger than me. She was a tireless breast cancer advocate and then she developed a very aggressive form of breast cancer herself, and she ultimately died. She left behind a young daughter and a husband. That was probably one of the toughest times for me, and that's when I really drew on the strength of friends who were also other physicians. They helped me rebalance the roles of friend and physician, which sometimes can be hard to play.

Dealing with bad outcomes is part of the reason why I've always done something else, so I wasn't fulltime in the clinic. I was never hit time after time after time with the 'giving the bad news' scenario. It's also why I did radiation oncology rather than medical oncology. I think that the MedOncs typically are doing more end-of-life care whereas, in my practice, even if I'm doing things palliatively for people toward the end of their lives, I'm not right there in that death and dying moment. I think that specialty would have put me at more risk of burnout.

Now that the kids are gone, exercise is a major coping mechanism for me and I try to walk every night. I try to always do things to disconnect. I read, but not anything that has any socially redeeming value. [*Laugh*] I read murder mysteries and crime novels and other things that are just totally fiction and take me to a different place, even if it is only for five or ten minutes a night. And my present husband isn't in medicine. He just retired from law enforcement and now teaches fulltime. He is a great person, and really, we get along well. We're very well-matched, and the kids love him. It's a very easy relationship.

Sometimes you go through hard things in life and think that the end of the world is coming. Then, later, you look back and realize that there was a purpose to it all. For me, everything wound up much better than I would have ever imagined. But when you are in that dark tunnel, you can't see the bright light in the future. It's a lesson that I've learned over time that I try to impart to my kids: it may look really dark or bleak now, but you just ride through it and things can turn out much better!

## Discussion or Writing Prompts

1  "There's a lot of guilt with trying to juggle work and motherhood." What are your struggles with integrating domestic, non-work activities, and work or school. When does a conflict arise and how do you resolve that?
2  Describe your own experiences with dual career relationships, either your own or those of someone close to you. What happens when one person achieves more "success?" How do gender roles impact the dynamic?
3  What strategies do you use to disconnect from medicine? Does it help to connect to people outside medicine? When do you prefer to connect with colleagues or classmates outside work or school?
4  Describe your journey with insecurities at work. Do they lessen over time, and if so, what accounts for that?
5  "In medicine, there's sometimes what I call a 'boot-camp mentality,' where it's like, 'Well, I've done it, and you should do it too.'" Describe the culture of your work or school environment. When do long hours, hard work, and sacrifice make sense and when do they lead to burnout or unnecessary distress?
6  "But giving bad news is a strain. Over time, you get better at doing it... after a while, you find a way of insulating yourself." Recall a time when you had to share bad news with a patient. How do you remain empathetic and self-protective?
7  How have you coped when a patient had a bad outcome?
8  Discuss a painful time in your life that in retrospect led to growth or opportunity.

# 18  Motherhood in Training

*Dr Cindy Volta is a primary care physician in her mid 30s who is deeply in touch with her emotions and memories. She discusses the importance of pregnancy planning and breastfeeding whilst working long shifts as an intern, and the later, devastating loss of another baby.*

I had my son right before I started my intern year of residency. He was only six weeks old, and we still had 30-hour calls. I was in the hospital a lot.

I was adamant that even though I couldn't be with him all the time, I would breastfeed or give him breast milk until he was a year old. I was also determined that being a new mom wouldn't impact my ability to be a good doctor and one of the top in my class. It was a lot of stress to put on myself, but I felt that that was the only way to be happy with my work.

I carried my breast pump every day on the wards and would be as efficient as possible in seeing my patients so I could run up and pump for 10–15 minutes before rounds. Then right before lunch and again in the afternoon, I'd pump.

My co-interns, residents, chiefs, and everyone on the program were awesome; so supportive! I can remember a few saying, "If you want me to see one of your patients, I'll go, so you can stay and pump." My husband was amazing as well.

I remember being on-call at two o'clock in the morning trying to pump and being so anxious about my patient who's in AFib. I can't break her rhythm, and she's getting sicker. I sat down pumping for ten minutes and I didn't have any milk let-down. I just got more and more frustrated and had to call my husband. He put the phone next to my son [*laughs*] and that helped give me let down. And that sort of thing happened on several occasions. But I made it a year and my son is now a big, healthy seven-year-old!

My husband and I got married before medical school. We kept trying to figure out the best time to have babies and there never seemed a perfect time. Towards the end of medical school, we're like, "Oh, this is probably a good time." We tried for nine months.

I found out I was pregnant when I was on an away rotation in San Francisco, so I wasn't even with him then. It was the day I was submitting my residency applications. We thought we would probably go somewhere outside

DOI: 10.4324/9781003475170-23

Texas because I was born and raised there. That changed once we found out we were pregnant. We wanted to minimize obstacles that would make it even more challenging to care for a newborn during intern year, so we chose to stay near our parents.

I had my second child, my daughter, when I was a chief resident. I did a chief because I love medical education and wanted to focus on that aspect of my career. There was more flexibility with the job, so I had my second baby that year.

Since I finished my training and started working as faculty, my work and homelife balance is much better. There are always the struggles of having to work later than expected and still having to pick up my kids, but it's definitely better than [*laugh*] how it was at the beginning.

But very sadly, my pregnancies weren't all straightforward. I'll probably cry thinking about it, but I did lose a baby in between my son and my daughter. That was probably the hardest thing that's happened to me. It still makes me so emotional!

I got pregnant during my third year of residency. I was doing a rotation away in Austin, so that delayed doing my anatomy scan for my baby until I was 23 weeks. She had a lot of deformities, and we ended up having to make some tough decisions. That was hard because with a second pregnancy you start showing so much earlier and everybody knew I was pregnant. Scheduling a pregnancy and a delivery in residency is a hard thing to do; we had already redone all the schedules and people were covering for me in times when I would be giving birth.

I was on a busy rotation, but again, my co-residents and my attending and the entire program were fantastic and helped me do what I had to do. My best friend from medical school is a neonatal intensive care doctor, so she was familiar with what my baby had. She called me and said, "Come to my hospital," which is the leading hospital in the United States for this disorder.

She hosted us in her house and helped us through all of that. Everybody else took care of our patients in the hospital and my parents stepped in to watch our son. We had just beautiful support, but obviously, it's still hard thinking about the loss. It makes me really treasure our two living babies.

Afterwards, it was really difficult figuring out how to go back to work. I would run into people months later, and they'd be like, "How's your baby?" I had to retell the story so many times, though it definitely got easier to tell.

Losing my baby has absolutely changed the way I relate to patients. It's important to figure out if you want to have babies at some point, and if you do, when to have them. We're so good at saying, "That would never happen to me. I'm going to have healthy kids, and everything's going to be OK." Now I counsel female patients about their reproductive plans.

If you are a professional female, that often means you're going to have babies later and you run more of a risk of having spontaneous deformities, or Down's, and things like that. Or pregnancy may not happen, or there may be some complication of pregnancy to your health. I guess I'd never thought about that when I started childbearing, which seems silly. Being a physician, you learn about all that stuff.

We also did a study with college students to see if they knew about and were creating their own reproductive life plans. Not a lot of women had thought about it. They were excellent at answering questions about their career goals but hadn't thought about if they wanted to get pregnant and what it would mean if they delayed pregnancy. The lesson to us as primary care physicians is that it is important to review this with our patients, so that they have all the information.

October 15 is National Pregnancy and Infant Loss Day for women who have had miscarriages or other pregnancy complications. I posted something on my Facebook about it. My husband saw it and he's like, "Oh, what was that?" I told him. He's like, "You still think about that?" I was like, "Of course, I do." In his mind, we'd moved on. We had a beautiful, healthy daughter after that. But I do still think about it, maybe because I take care of women. I talk about their gynecological history, and I recognize how common it is to have pregnancy complications. A loss is hard. It can shape who you are. It has for me.

---

### Discussion or Writing Prompts

1  "We kept trying to figure out the best time to have babies and there never seemed a perfect time." Recall a scenario from your life in which you were challenged to plan for a family or a significant personal event requiring you to take a leave of absence. Describe your emotions in response to the dilemma.

2  At which stage in your training or career do you think it would be best to have a baby? Discuss the pros and cons of considering a reproductive plan and the implications for yourself or someone you care about.

3  "He put the phone next to my son [*Laugh*] and that helped give me let down." How do you manage the stress of feeling split between being with a patient and being with your family?

4  "Losing my baby has absolutely changed the way I relate to patients." Describe how a personal experience changed how you relate to patients.

# 19  Regrets and Dedication

*Dr Grace Lakeland has encountered racism and sexism and could never find the right time to have children. Now she mentors younger women throughout her hospital system, giving them the sort of support that she once desperately needed.*

I am a general surgeon, practicing for about 15 years now. I love surgery because it's a team sport. You travel around in a pack, you make decisions as a team, it's like when I played sports growing up and traveled around with the team working really, really hard.

But my surgery training was very difficult. While there were some women in surgical residency, there were significantly fewer than there are now. There were four open positions a year in my program and in my year the universe somehow produced four women for those spots. And I was the first black woman. We were very happy, thinking we had found our passions, but the Chair of Surgery was awful. He would make comments in front of other people, such as "Is this a gynecology program?" He also shared that there was once a black male resident in the program and he would never match another because he was "lazy." I am not sure if that was supposed to be a warning or not to me!

Whenever I went to see the Chair, he made me sit outside his office on the floor! He would smoke in there, because back then, they would smoke in the office. He never, never acknowledged me.

I just felt like I needed to finish the program, but that I wouldn't practice surgery when I was done. My husband remembers that I used to say all the time, "If this is how I have to live for the rest of my career, I won't do it." But I didn't want to quit the training and prove them right in thinking that I couldn't make it.

Well, I am still practicing surgery! I'm the only one of the four women who went into the training program that stayed in the field.

I don't know why that Chair of Surgery behaved so terribly. It was my very first year and you're just a fledgling at that point, working very hard. You feel like no one really acknowledges you; that you're this "scut monkey," is what we called it. You feel like you're not quite as worthy as the other residents. My whole training period was just very dark!

DOI: 10.4324/9781003475170-24

At the time, I thought it was because I was a first-year resident; I am the type of person to try to find other reasons outside of race and gender for mistreatment. But now I see clearly it was because I am a woman. In the past five years, that man was fired due to sexism and a variety of things that come with that.

Now I have a senior position in the hospital—I've finally made it. I have a PhD and an MBA, I'm boarded in both critical care and general surgery. At the last American College of Surgeons' meeting, I went up to him and told him what I was doing. I thought he'd be happy, but he wasn't. I left the dinner. [*Laugh*] I was very disappointed, but you can't find your happiness in one person, and I'm a very happy person!

I didn't have a mentor going through my training period but now I mentor female physicians, nurse practitioners and medical students. I'm leading the general surgery interest group for the medical school, just so people can have a voice, and say, "Am I feeling this way for this reason?" Sometimes the reasons concern patients. We may make poor judgments and then things go wrong, which is even worse than people failing to respond to our therapy. Those times never leave you; they scar your soul. And man, many times, things go wrong despite our best efforts.

It's never been easy for me; I've always had to fight a little bit, but I don't see myself as unique because everyone in the healthcare field has had to work hard and make sacrifices. But I get comments constantly because people think that I've had some advantages because I'm a woman and I'm not Caucasian. They assume that I'm in my position not because of my hard work and training, but because I meet some certain quota. It's a bit distressing, but you just prove them wrong.

My best friend here is another surgeon, also very successful. She was training underneath me when we first started on critical care. She would come in at five o'clock in the morning and I would be there. Then she came in at four o'clock in morning and I'd be there. Then she was like, "That's it. I'm not coming in any earlier." [*Laugh*] I used to go to work at 3:30 in the morning, and other people have very similar stories; it was psychologically awful!

The limit right now during training is 80 hours a week. Before that, we used to work over 100 hours a week. [*Laugh*] It definitely was not safe for patients! I remember I would walk into my house, drop all my clothes at the door and go to bed. Then I would get up and go to work at 3 o'clock in the morning!

It was extremely stressful and unhealthy. You don't eat well; you start gaining weight. I don't know if you really think clearly. Also I had problems with anxiety and a little bit of depression then.

Now I probably work 60–80 hours a week and do 12-hour shifts over the weekend. I won't do more than three nights in a row because I don't think clearly. I think the healthcare field self-selects the people that can work those long hours. In the surgical field, when you perform a procedure, it's very difficult to leave the patient in the hands of someone who wasn't there. Changing providers all the time is linked to higher complications and mortality because you can't easily convey some types of information during the hand-off. Everyone everywhere has been struggling with that.

In some specialties it's easier, certainly. If people want to have a family, then perhaps they won't choose a specialty where they're working 80 hours a week or doing nights on the weekend. I've had to sacrifice; I don't have children, there was no time. I have regrets, I always will!

This is one of the things that I advise women about, and especially the medical students who ask, "When is it the right time to have a child?" Do they do it in medical school when they're studying all the time? Is it something you do in your first residency year when you're trying to make a name for yourself? Is it OK to have a baby when you get a job, or will everyone look at you and say, "Well, that person isn't going to pull their weight, because they're going to want to go home?"

I tell them there's never a good time. You just must do it when you feel it's right. I delayed it, and then I couldn't have children anymore. It's really important that people are very mindful along the way.

Though I don't have children, I have many other things that fulfill my life. I do a lot of charity work: I just got back from Haiti where we did 80 surgeries. I started going there in 2011, after the earthquake, and I've been a couple of times a year since then. It gives me focus and resilience and makes me realize where my priorities lie, but basically, I go there to serve other people and it feels like the right thing to do. I have a friend who says that we are pampered American poodles in a world of wolves!

When we started going to Haiti there was no hospital, just tents and shipping containers and we put in beds and hung IV poles. Next there were plywood walls and finally, many years after the earthquake, we opened the hospital. But in the early days we couldn't provide the type of basic care that we have here in the United States. I remember a 19-year-old boy coming in with an asthma attack and there was no ventilator in the hospital. We put a breathing tube in his airway and manually bagged him and tried to break his asthma attack, but he died, and that just doesn't happen in first-world countries. He died! Then we had to put him in a body bag and take him to the morgue and the following morning we buried him. We barely had a ceremony for him.

Those type of things matter to me. Certainly, I've had a lot of struggles in the past but sometimes they don't feel very real, as if I'm making a big deal out of nothing. Maybe I forget them because they're not as large as the struggle faced by the mother of that boy. She was there the whole time and so thankful. Can you imagine? So thankful because she knew that we did everything in our power to help him. So that's what is important to me now.

**Writing or Discussion Prompts**

1 How would you feel when being devalued or humiliated at work or in training. How would you cope? How can such behavior be stopped?

2 Describe strategies to recognize and constructively respond to sexual discrimination, whether subtle or explicit.

3 Dr Lakeland describes constantly having to prove herself because of assumptions about African Americans' qualifications. How would you feel if colleagues or patients were silently or overtly questioning your worthiness?

4 Discuss the impact on health and the trade-offs associated with excessive work during training.

5 "I've had to sacrifice; I don't have children, there was no time. I have regrets. I always will!" Explore your reactions. What should be done to support parental leave during surgery training?

6 Describe how you find meaning or fulfillment outside work.

7 Describe how you think you would cope with being responsible for a bad outcome of a patient. What kinds of support would benefit the emotional fallout?

8 Explore your emotional response to hearing the story of the boy in impoverished Haiti dying for lack of a ventilator, yet his mother was grateful to the medical staff for trying to save him.

# Part VI

# COVID-19

# 20 Family Life in COVID Times

*Dr Isabella Austin is a Mexican American gastroenterologist and a transplant hepatology fellow in a large teaching hospital. As with so many other physicians, life became very difficult when COVID-19 reached her city. She is talking here in late 2020, less than a year into the pandemic.*

I was born and raised in Mexico and obtained my medical degree there. When I was finishing my first year of general surgery, I realized that I really enjoyed the gastrointestinal part, but I missed the patient interaction. Even though I love Mexico and have a lot of family and very dear friends there, I knew that I wanted something different. The United States is one of the best places to study to become a physician, so I moved to the United States, literally with nothing. I needed to re-qualify as a physician, even though I was already doing general surgery in Mexico.

It was really challenging because I couldn't just sit down and study. I needed to support myself and I was very lucky to find a part-time job as a research coordinator in hepatology at a top university. I worked there for two years and that's where I became interested in liver disease. I had amazing mentors that I'm still in touch with and they keep pushing me. I'm very grateful for all the people that I've met throughout this path!

I took my exams to qualify as a physician in the United States and then matched to do internal medicine on the East Coast. I did three years of internal medicine, and then an extra year as a chief resident and then matched here. It's been a very long road! Meanwhile, I got married and my husband is my biggest supporter and cheerleader. He's amazing. He works from home and is happy to move anywhere. I just couldn't do what I do if it wasn't for him!

When COVID-19 arrived, there was a lot of stuff that we didn't know about it. We had to think, "How do you maintain social distancing? What are the different precautions we need to take in the hospital? When do we need to use PPE (personal protection equipment)? And driving home, what are the measures I need to take before I see my family?" I have two girls under four years old, so it's been quite challenging. I'm very grateful and lucky to have a lot of support at home from my husband and my mom, who is living with us,

DOI: 10.4324/9781003475170-26

which obviously has its pros and cons because she's elderly and that puts her at high risk for COVID.

When COVID arrived in this State, I was just about to begin a month of service and would be in contact with patients that could be COVID positive and maybe asymptomatic and I was thinking, "What if I pass on the virus?" It was really, really hard. So, as a family, we decided it would be safer if I isolated from all my family for the month and moved to a separate house.

I remember arriving at this random house I'd rented. I'm crying my eyes out because I wasn't going to see my daughters, husband, and Mama for weeks. My youngest was almost seven months old and my eldest was two, super little! The youngest was okay because she didn't really know what was going on and she just smiled. But my almost three-year-old struggled, constantly asking "Where's Mami?" She calls me Mami because I'm from Mexico. And every day my husband was sending me videos of her and my other daughter and leaving notes outside the house where I was living. It was just heartbreaking. And I was working crazy hours as well, at least 12-hour shifts, even during the weekends, and treating COVID-19 patients in very cumbersome health situations.

My two daughters, my husband, and my mom were just completely isolated, and I was the only one having contact with the outside world, doing the groceries. Every time that I used to drop off the groceries, my almost three-year-old would be banging on the window, because she's seeing me outside the glass and screaming and I'm just crying my eyes out. That's the only interaction I had with my daughters in a month. We have this video of me delivering the groceries that still makes me teary when I see it. It also makes me value little things.

Before leaving for my COVID house, I'd been breastfeeding my baby. That's a hard point: I actually had to stop. It was really, really hard because I breastfed my first daughter for a year, and with Ella, my little one, I was only able to breastfeed her for six months before I had to leave her. Stopping that was a very difficult decision. I still feel guilt, because I gave the opportunity to one daughter and not to the other, but as a fellow, with COVID going on, it was just too dangerous to be living with them.

After a month I returned to my children. Oh my God—it was amazing! I'll never forget that day! It was my three-year-old daughter Jasmine's birthday, and we delayed her birthday for a week without her knowing! I hid in a big box and my husband told her, "Hey, your birthday gift, it's outside." And then she came outside and opened the box and I was inside. It was crazy!

Even now when I come home from work I have a little routine. Nobody else is allowed to get into my car, ever. In my garage I close the door, strip off, drop my clothes in the washing machine—the shoes stay outside—and then I just go straight into the shower. And now my three-year-old knows that after Mama has her shower, she's allowed to come and hug and kiss me.

It was a very scary situation. We weren't sure of the precautions we needed to take. And what if I got infected? Even a couple of weeks ago, I got an upper respiratory infection from one of my daughters and I was freaking out because I started having a little bit of chest pain, shortness of breath, and a sore throat. I was like, "Oh my God, I have COVID!" So, you start thinking about all the things that could happen, especially to my mom. It would just break my heart if I, as the high-risk person, passed on COVID. I worry not only for my mom but also for my daughters and my husband.

In those early days, people didn't know what to do with COVID patients. It was very quiet at the beginning, but we were all scared and worried because we were hearing what was happening in New York, and we had this big expectation of having a huge surge here. And it was really challenging because as gastroenterologists, we do endoscopies and colonoscopies, and you need to take special precautions with those as well. And the guidelines and recommendations were changing every day. So, one day it's like, "Oh, you don't need to wear masks." And then next day it's like, "Oh, you actually need to wear a mask." And now it's, "You don't just need a mask, you need to wear an N-95 mask." Also, we didn't know if we were going to have enough PPE, and because of wanting to save PPE—and I think this was the right decision— they canceled procedures or stopped us trainees performing any procedures, and that's one of the things that I enjoy most about my specialty. I didn't know how all this would affect my training, because you only have three years to train. And I was just going back at night to my "COVID house" as I called it, not knowing how long I was going to have to stay isolated from my family. It wasn't fun but I learned a lot from that experience.

Thousands of people have died of COVID in this part of our State. We've had a high number of COVID patients at my hospital and the problem is that some of them don't get discharged for months and months. We have a lot of patients right now that have been here for three, four, or five months. We did have a surge but not as big as in many other places. I feel that our hospital did a great job to prepare for the unexpected and for the worst. They created groups to be ready to cover for other physicians. For example, in my case, even though I am a gastroenterology and a transplant hepatology fellow, I was part of the emergency department surge. So, if they wanted some backup, I was ready to go to help with consults and do whatever was needed. There are even attendings right now from gastroenterology and hepatology that are still in surge standby, just in case.

It is really hard for the patients too, especially because they are isolated and just seeing all these masks or screens, without being able to have much one-to-one interaction with the medical staff. I try to find ways to make it a little bit easier for them; I kind of joke around and show them the picture on my ID to try to make things a little more personal. I have some Latino patients with other conditions and sometimes COVID too. I remember one very well—she was a patient with a new diagnosis of cancer. We had to perform an endoscopic procedure and we couldn't make a human connection with her because of the masks. So, I spoke in Spanish to her—that's what I normally do whenever I see a patient that I know hasn't got English as their native language, and I feel that it definitely gives them a little bit of peace in some way. And then, unfortunately, she tested positive for COVID. Thank God she did well, but it delayed her cancer diagnosis and treatment and, of course, she needed to be isolated from everyone. But the ones that I've seen in the ICU are unfortunately very, very sick. Most of them are intubated. Luckily, I've seen several patients that I started following months ago who are now extubated and recovering from this horrible disease, which is very gratifying.

I felt very supported by everyone in my program. The hospital created a lot of coping strategies and tried to do social activities online to keep our spirits up, because it was such a difficult time for everyone. I obviously didn't go public and tell everyone that I was isolating myself, but the people I told were very supportive and helped me in every way. I even got gifts—a ton of stuff sent to my "COVID house," and constant emails and text messages: "How are you doing? You're a trooper, keep going."

The whole COVID experience has been a huge learning experience, from a personal and a professional perspective. I'm the one going out and working at the hospital, but my husband is the one staying with my daughters and keeping our house afloat. He is my rock and this whole experience has brought us even closer. It's brought not only my family closer, but also my colleagues and co-fellows and attendees, because we shared and showed different kinds of vulnerabilities, and it's given us a lot of growth opportunities. And best of all, all my colleagues and people who are close to me and have gotten COVID are okay. But it's certainly been challenging, for sure!

## Discussion or Writing Prompts

1  Think about how much of a calling medicine is for foreign medical graduates who overcome years of retraining, exams, and adjusting to a new medical system and culture. What makes your career path a calling and how much might you be willing to endure for it.

2  Due to isolating from her family in order to treat patients, Dr Austin had to stop breast-feeding six months earlier than planned. Think about what sustained her during this time. Discuss a difficult trade-off that you've had to make. What sustained you?

3  "We have this video of me delivering the groceries that still makes me teary when I see it. It also makes me value little things." What do you not want to take for granted? How can you sustain your appreciation and gratitude for it?

4 Discuss your work/homelife balance with or without a supportive partner. What are some ways to get the help needed at home and support for your professional life?
5 Explore a situation that you were suddenly thrown into without preparation, or with a lot of uncertainty and fear. How did you manage? What helped you cope, or what might have helped you cope better?
6 "....we couldn't make a human connection with her because of the masks. So, I spoke in Spanish to her." Describe a time that you overcame a barrier with a patient due to some shared human connection.
7 Describe the ways you have felt supported by your program/department/colleagues during a stressful time. Or conversely, the impact on you when they failed to provide support.

# 21   The COVID-19 Experience

*Dr John Sutton is a young physician who was supervising a large team of junior doctors when the COVID-19 pandemic first hit the major cities of the United States. He describes living through those terrifying, chaotic days and making life and death decisions based on sketchy information.*

I came to America from Canada just before my 18th birthday to attend university on a tennis scholarship and afterward I had a go at playing professionally. Then, for reasons including injury, I pursued medicine as a career. I went to medical school out east and then worked in the health system in Philadelphia. I was a board-certified internal medicine doctor, working as an attending, completely independently. My program had kind of a unique role, so I was a chief resident overseeing the internal medicine residency program and above me were the assistant program director and the program director. And I also worked as a hospitalist and cross-covered the intensive care unit.

I got married three years ago; we met at medical school seven years prior. My wife was a year behind me in schooling, so I did an extra year to get us on track together so that when we moved somewhere, we wouldn't be separated.

I was working in the hospital in Philadelphia as the pandemic hit. And the challenges, not just for me but also for my friends and my wife, were profound. My wife had to work in the intensive care unit during nights; this is when we were all figuring out how to cope. A lot of the things we went through then definitely led to trauma and dark days. We had some very difficult times in those first few months. We were looking after very, very sick patients.

When we first heard about COVID, we were just like anyone else, but then we got immersed in it. The other chief resident (a pulmonary critical care fellow) and I were responsible for 65 other residents, overseeing their schedules and dealing with sickness. We really had no idea what to expect. We saw what was happening in China and Italy and assumed the worst. We were making changes to people's schedules, telling them that they couldn't go on vacation, visit family members, go to weddings and birthdays and we, of course, were sacrificing those same things ourselves.

DOI: 10.4324/9781003475170-27

We would be calling people out: "Hey, we need extra help tonight. You're gonna have to come in and work a shift in the ICU." And at that time, at the beginning, the hospital policy was that we were only allowed to wear masks in the patient's rooms and not in the hallway. So we would put on a mask, throw it in the trash, walk to the next patient's room, pick up a mask and put it on. And we weren't allowed to wear masks in the cafeteria. Obviously, later there was a complete 180-degree change about that.

I remember giving a talk with the other chief resident to our hospital medicine group; I pulled up all the COVID information out there. It felt like there were new updates coming out of Italy and China daily, things they'd learnt, things they were learning. At the beginning, the data was all about using hydroxychloroquine and not using steroids. I remember recommending that regime to our group. We also recommended early mechanical ventilation. We weren't using non-invasive measures like C-PAP and bi-level ventilation, like the external masks, because we were worried about aerosolization of the virus. We were putting people on ventilators when they were getting to about six liters of oxygen, and that was based on data coming out of one of the top hospitals on the east coast. They put out a kind of handbook about it. Also, I think it was based on reports from Italy saying that once people got to six liters, they rapidly progressed to respiratory failure, so it was better to ventilate them early on.

We were trying to get hold of PPE (personal protective equipment) at that time, and we didn't have adequate testing. We were waiting seven, ten days to get a test back. So, a patient would come in and we were looking at their laboratory values, low lymphocyte counts and things like that, which may point to them having COVID. That's how we were deciding to intubate them. Then maybe they would go up to the intensive care unit and die, and then we would get the COVID test back. Sometimes it was negative. By intubating that patient, did we hasten their death in any way? I guess we won't ever really know. It was just an incredible time to practice medicine.

But I definitely felt responsible if people did badly and died. I think everybody did. We had a system in our hospital to protect the health care workers. When somebody had a cardiac arrest and they had COVID or suspected COVID, a code blue 19 was called. Everyone knew that when they got to the room, they had to put on a gown and a mask and proper PPE equipment. You could see the patient wasn't breathing and their heart had stopped, but you couldn't go in the room; you had to protect yourself. But it goes against everything you've trained for, to stand outside the room and watch someone die in front of you and not be able to do anything. There were a number of occasions like that.

There was a lot of death and dying and we weren't allowing visitors to patients. We had patients who just died in the hospital, completely alone. If I was on that night, I'd go and sit in the room with them just so they weren't alone. Families could only say goodbye by FaceTime. It was something I'll never forget. We definitely weren't trained for this. Certainly, it was a duty, but it was something that was really difficult to be involved with, and something I don't think we'll ever experience again. Sometimes we had doctors on a night-time shift who were only 26, 27 years old. And nurses, even younger, would do the same thing.

We had whole families, grandparents and kids, that I admitted to the hospital at the same time. I think the worst I remember was an elderly patient in her early eighties who had COVID. We had the conversation with her that if things got bad and she was heading toward having to go on a ventilator, that she should consider, um, you know, less aggressive means. Because what we've seen is that patients that progressed this way at her age, with her type of morbidities, generally don't come off the ventilator. And the family was very understanding. The daughter was a doctor and they asked if they could come in and say goodbye to the mother. And that was the time we had the strictest rules—we eventually eased up a little bit once the cases came down. But I had to tell her, "No, you can't come in and see her." She had to FaceTime. She said goodbye to her mother as I'm sitting in the room, and then her mother passed shortly afterward. But I felt I had no place being there during that moment between that family. I'm a complete stranger, telling her she can't come in and see her dying mother. I'm sure she remembers that vividly, as I do.

It was the worst, most terrifying situation for everyone, for myself and my wife and for all my friends too. It was the anticipatory dread of going into work. You just had no idea if it was going to be one of those jam-packed nights where you don't stop moving for 12 hours, with people dying all around you. I mean, it was terrible. I will give kudos to our hospital system. They did a good job supporting us and my boss was really in tune to the burnout that was taking place. We all completely rearranged our schedules, with the buy-in of everyone, so at least we were getting some breaks. But it was terrible because you would basically go home, immediately strip off at the front door, put your clothes in a bag, jump in the shower, wash your clothes, go to bed exhausted and then get up and do the same the next day. And it went on and on for months. It was honestly kind of blurring. It seems like the time went by so fast, but it took so long as well.

It was the most eventful year of my life, for sure; very intense emotionally. Both my wife and I had symptoms, and both got tested and were negative, so I guess we avoided it. We had friends and colleagues who tested positive and got sick. Some of them got quite ill. I have friends at other hospitals who've had co-workers die. We consider ourselves lucky from the standpoint that we never got it. None of my co-workers that I know personally died from it, but a lot of people on the periphery got sick and unfortunately some of them passed away, which is just, you know, unthinkable.

**Discussion or Writing Prompts**

1  "A lot of the things we went through then definitely led to trauma and dark days." Discuss a time when you were thrown into a stressful clinical situation where you did not feel prepared.

2  What helped medical workers cope in the early days of the pandemic when they were witnessing frequent deaths, working exhausting shifts, and forgoing vacation time?

3  Describe how you would resolve conflict over treatment options when the best form of treatment is not yet known.

4  What would your emotional reaction be if you discovered that a colleague had become ill or died as a result of practicing medicine?

5  "But I definitely felt responsible if people did badly and died." How would you support a colleague in this situation?

# 22 COVID-19, the Aftermath

*Dr Sutton was a board-certified internal medicine physician in charge of a large team of junior doctors in a Philadelphia hospital when the COVID-19 pandemic first hit the major cities of the United States. He worked nonstop through those terrifying, chaotic days, making life and death decisions based on sketchy information and little sleep. In Fall 2020, he began retraining as a hematologist. However, he was unprepared for the burnout he felt.*

I'm now in my fifth year of being a doctor. I've moved to the southwest from Philadelphia and left internal medicine for hematology, the field I really want to be in. It's been a roundabout way to get here! I think the hardest transition was going back to being the junior doctor, an intern again. Now, quite rightly, I'm having oversight while learning a whole new field of medicine. It feels good though!

When I started here and had a bit of downtime and the intensity was lower, I really struggled with feelings of depression and anxiety and burnout. In my first month I seriously considered quitting my hematology fellowship and taking time off because I was just so burned out from what had just happened. I hadn't really had time to think about what we'd gone through, because just as things were starting to get better with COVID-19 numbers going down in Philadelphia, we moved to the other side of the country. I remember when we first came down here, we couldn't believe that the cities hadn't had a real lockdown and didn't even require anyone to wear a mask!

We were like, "This is just the most ignorant thing imaginable!" We were so mad about that because we had just been through the terrible situation in Philadelphia. That definitely contributed to my feelings of burnout and I really considered transitioning away from medicine. Now we know COVID is here to stay, but we have vaccines and cases are way, way down and much better treated, so I'm hopeful for the future. If COVID returned badly again, I would feel obligated to volunteer to help because I think my experience from the first-time round in Philadelphia would be useful. But at the same time, I don't want to.

Even my marriage was affected during the time working with COVID patients. Our relationship is very strong; we can sit next to each other and

DOI: 10.4324/9781003475170-28

not need to talk, but we were just shorter with each other because we were exhausted. When the other person walked in the door, you never knew what kind of day they'd had. I noticed that several relationships in the medical field, not just marriages, but engagements, broke up during or shortly after it. But we are very happy now—things are great. We just found out that we're pregnant!

What I'm doing now, hematology oncology, is a big commitment. It's three extra years of training when I could have gone out and made a real salary, but it's something I've always wanted to do. I've personally had a melanoma—skin cancer. I got diagnosed the day I picked up my moving truck to drive to medical school. I got a phone call because I'd had a biopsy. Up until that point, I wanted to do orthopedic surgery because I played tennis and sports, but after that melanoma, I became fascinated by cancer care.

My work in hematology is mostly outpatient, so it should be a little more relaxed than in some branches of medicine. That's part of my reasoning when considering what to do for a career choice. However, going into training, I underestimated the emotional toll of seeing patients with end-stage cancer. If they've got pancreatic cancer, for instance, you know only 50% are going to be alive in one year. I think that was another reason why, at the beginning of this fellowship, I was like, "I'm not sure I can do this, see all this death and dying all the time." I was feeling so beaten down by the death and dying we saw with COVID in Philadelphia. But as I've gone through my training here, I've seen some people do well and come out the other side. And in the attending clinic or working with some of the senior consultants, I've seen patients coming back that are five years out and doing well and just returning for a social, "How are you doing?" type of check-up.

So, you know, I think there's a different side to it. If you can find a good therapy or a clinical trial for patients to go on, you're helping them have extra quality time that they wouldn't otherwise have. I think that shift in my thinking has been helpful.

However, I still feel quite pressured and I've looked into doing therapy. I know my employer has resources to help but it feels somehow wrong to seek help through your employer, I don't know why. It's not distrust, but I just would like to keep it separate. My wife is an outpatient internal medicine doctor here and I lean on her a lot, which is healthy? Unhealthy? Probably a bit of both! But I think there's a big stigma around mental health in general and especially in medicine. You can't ever admit that you're struggling with anything.

I actually did reach out to my associate program director here though. I said, "Hey, look, I'm really struggling right now. I need a break or something because I can't continue like this." She, to her credit, was nothing but helpful, listening and offering resources. We tweaked my schedule and added in an extra month of research, which I'm on right now, just to give me a little more of a break.

It's taking time to get over that intense COVID experience, I'm still feeling burned out. And with all the transitions, I've never really had a time to process what happened, but I feel in a better place right now. I still have bad days when I'm not sure that this is what I want to do, though I think that pretty much every trainee in America has similar feelings at some point. Not to mean that it should be normalized, I just think it's something that goes with the career right now.

I've worked very hard to get where I am, but I'm a doctor and I recognize that I'm privileged. I know I could be much worse off!

## Discussion or Writing Prompts

1 "...when we first came down here, we couldn't believe that the cities hadn't had a real lockdown and didn't even require anyone to wear a mask!" Describe a time you struggled to empathize with a patient who held different views than your own.

2 Consider a time that your work took a toll on your outside relationships. What kinds of things can be done to sustain a relationship during and alongside the early years of a career in medicine?

3 Describe a time when you or a peer were struggling emotionally. What were the barriers to asking for help? What facilitates help-seeking? How do you feel about seeking therapy through your employer?

4 How do you identify your right career path and professional identity?

5 "You can't ever admit that you're struggling with anything." What can program directors or leaders do to make it easier to acknowledge emotional distress?

# Part VII
# Burnout

# 23 Leadership

*Dr Richard Brady was Senior Vice-President for Clinical Operations at a large non-profit nursing home system in the Northeast that specialized in end-of-life care. As the homes multiplied to serve the needs of the city's expanding population, he pulled 13–14-hour days, 6 days a week, sacrificing family time for the care of his dying patients. Eventually poor leadership at the top of the organization caused him to resign. He's still overcoming the trauma of it all.*

I was brought on by an executive director who was wonderful and her body of work, over time, is exceptional. We worked very closely for about 20 years; she allowed me to grow, gave me huge responsibility, paid me extremely well and I owe my entire career to her. But she was a difficult personality.

I started clinically, but then in the last ten years I evolved to be one of the two senior leaders and ran all the clinical operations, and eventually I became the senior vice-president.

We were a small organization that got huge. Laurie, who reported directly to me, was one of the best people I've ever worked with. He was respected, charismatic, organized, detailed, educated, thirsty to learn, a good person. I really connected with him, mentoring and coaching him. We were a great team. Then his life spun out of control, personally and professionally, and he died by suicide.

I didn't know a whole lot about his personal life until after he killed himself. We didn't always have a lot of time to discuss stuff because we were very busy. It turned out that he was a complicated person, a kind of Jekyll and Hyde character. Outside work he was very disorganized. He took financial risks, had relationship problems, was a philanderer, probably into some drugs. The professional persona was just the opposite. It's so unfortunate how the personal part of his life spun out of control. I felt deep hurt when he died.

When Laurie killed himself, we had to reorganize, and I had to start over and form a different leadership team. Laurie basically oversaw all the end-of-life care we did. It was a huge role, and when he died, I took on all his responsibilities so the organization could save money. I did it because I love the organization and there was a need. I never stood back and said, "This is an impossible task for one person." I knew I could do it; the question is, how

DOI: 10.4324/9781003475170-30

well did I do it and at what cost? So physically and emotionally, I carried a lot more responsibility after Laurie's death, maybe too much.

I wasn't eating that well and I lost weight, and I stopped working out as much. I'd get up at 4:30 in the morning, be in the office by 6:00 am, and I'd work until 7:00 or 8:00 at night. I'd go in on a Saturday. My wife's a physician, so we'd always had limited time together, but now we had even less, and I have four children. I'm not a drinker or anything like that, but I sure wanted to be!

People started coming up to me saying, "You don't look good. [*Laugh*] You look really tired." I'd say "Yeah, we're all tired."

That organization draws in workers who don't always have good balance in their lives because they are so deeply committed to getting the end-of-life scenario right. If you do it wrong, the family is left with a nightmare for the rest of their lives. So everyone worked hard.

During those last few years without Laurie, I had a team of eight people and we did a lot of amazing things together, growing new programs. But eventually I had a little difficulty with the executive director. She was getting towards the end of her career and could no longer really understand the healthcare system. She'd become a long-standing legacy leader and didn't want to let go.

At the same time, the organization was involved in stressful financial change, and we were getting more competition from other types of elderly care facilities. All of that came together and we had our first-ever set of lay-offs. We did what we could to cope with the transitions, but several times people asked me to go to the board and basically try to oust the executive director. I refused to do that because it would have been messy and would totally have damaged the organization. And then people started to leave because it was just not good.

I probably should have spoken up sooner with her privately. I admit that several times she said that I abandoned her as a leader, which really meant she couldn't control me, but I've always felt that we need to be loyal to the mission, not to an individual. Part of the problem was that I would update her, but then she'd forget. She would come into my office, and say, "What the heck's going on?" I'd say, "We talked about this a month ago." Well, she didn't remember, so that was another challenge. If there is a lesson in all of this, I didn't learn it. [*Laugh*] I thought I was doing everything I could to be a team player.

But we all became disillusioned when we discovered a plan by the leader to appoint someone that she'd mentored, who wasn't a clinician, to replace her. She was not open to any outward search for the next executive director. When I started to speak up, she considered me disruptive and assumed I wanted her role, which I did not. I wanted an open search, instead of this secret deal. I just got more and more frustrated, and once I started losing section directors, I had to eventually say, "I'm done," and then I resigned. She couldn't believe it. I said, "No, it's time." When I left they replaced me with three people.

They wanted me to have a big farewell with the executive director able to say, "Everything's fine, Richard's just moving on." I said, "No. I'm not going out there to trash anyone, but I'm not going to smile." I was tired. I was done. I worked for a month after resigning and I said goodbye individually, but nothing big.

I was one of ten people who left the organization over a period of two years. It has now reorganized. But I was really angry that it lost such good people who knew where healthcare was going and knew about leadership development. We'd been moving in a great direction, but programs we'd started just died after we all left. I think I was angry that I couldn't fix it or make it work at the end. The facilities still give good patient care, I've used them. But many of us know that the organization would be a much better place and better positioned for the future if those wonderful people who resigned had stayed.

It's now 18 months since I left. It took me about a year to heal; to travel, spend time with family and recover. I would look in the mirror and see someone I didn't like, because I was becoming, out of my frustration, someone that just wasn't me.

After I recovered, I did have regrets about how I'd left. I'd worked so hard to be connected to the organization and to the people, and suddenly, I was gone. I've now reached back to the organization and met with the new executive director—the one that was first slipped into place when I was there only lasted about six months—and I'm getting involved again where I feel it would be helpful.

When I think back over the years, I see that I gave too much of myself. If you are going to work so hard for something you care about so deeply, you must go into it with your eyes wide open. You must talk to people you respect and love and get their opinion. You must be aware of the prices you'll pay and assess those along the way. But it wasn't all a mistake. I did a good job, and I really helped the organization get through a tough time, so overall I don't regret it. But now I'm happy and enjoying being involved in different things, instead of being in one position that almost buried me!

---

## Discussion and Writing Prompts

1 Why did Dr Brady feel "deep hurt" when his colleague died by suicide? Describe a time when you were unaware of a valued peer or colleague's personal suffering.

2 "When I think back over the years, I see that I gave too much of myself." Discuss working in a culture that requires you to go above and beyond. Is it hard to recognize your personal limits when you are fully committed to meaningful work?

3 "I've always felt that we need to be loyal to the mission, not to an individual." Consider a time when there was a contradiction

> between your values and those of a leader, peer, or institutional directive.
> 4   Have you witnessed good people leave your team or organization? What might have been done to retain them? Alternatively, consider a time when someone was planning to leave and they changed their mind. What helped them stay?

## Resource

American Foundation for Suicide Prevention. (n.d.). Support after suicide loss for healthcare professionals and organizations. https://afsp.org/support-after-suicide-loss-for-healthcare-professionals-and-organizations/.

# 24 The Pain Clinic Doctor's Despair

*Dr Angela Heredia is a mid-career pain specialist in private practice. She's been experiencing intense pressure from both her patients and practice owners to prescribe opioids against her better clinical judgment. She often encounters aggression from her patients and is weary with the continual battles she fights.*

After I graduated from medical school, I went into a residency in Physical Medicine & Rehabilitation. Then I moved here for a fellowship and I've been in a pain medicine private practice ever since.

When I chose this specialty, I felt that I was doing a service for people who had chronic and acute pain, and that chronic pain was misunderstood and undertreated. Now I find I'm prescribing a lot more opioids than I would like and I'm treating a lot more chronic pain than acute pain. I'm realizing that there are a lot of psychological overlays; I'm more of a therapist than a physician.

I only prescribe opioids to a small, select group of patients, who I feel are appropriate candidates. However, I would say that the majority of patients demand opioid medication and have been on it for years. They've tried other alternatives and I'm probably the fifth or sixth pain physician they've seen, and they don't want anything new.

After my first encounter with the patients, I see them at maybe their fourth or fifth visit. In between, they see my physician assistant or my nurse practitioner. They have been trained to just refill every month unless there's some change, or unless the patient violates the opioid agreement.

When the patient eventually sees me again, I try to introduce them to other pain medications that may treat their pain more effectively, but I've gotten the same negative response over and over again. It becomes more of an argument. I usually give in because I see that they're suffering. I feel their resistance to change and their fear. I want to alleviate that fear.

---

* (Note: This story was recorded before opioid prescribing was severely curtailed. Dr Heredia's laugh is not lighthearted—rather a reaction to the sadness of the situation. She is actually a little tearful.)

DOI: 10.4324/9781003475170-31

I feel like I'm hitting my head against the wall. My nurse practitioner and physician assistant don't want to have an argument with the patient either. I sit next to my PA and my NP and we work closely and have conversations about reducing the opioids. Sometimes those conversations are successful and sometimes they just give in to the patient.

I had a lot of complaints from patients early on in my career. I had a meeting with the administration who told me that I needed to change, that patients were complaining, and it wasn't about opioids. But they wouldn't give me examples of the complaints. Well, that, to me, was wrong, because how could I learn or know how to change my behavior?

To my mind, they didn't want to say what I really thought was going on, which was that they wanted me to prescribe opioids when the patients asked for them. Make the patients happy and not ruffle anybody's feathers.

I feel that I was doing the right thing by not refilling opioids. But I think over time, I've become the physician they wanted me to be, the one that makes the patient happy. Pain clinics thrive on chronic pain patients because they come in every month for their refills and that keeps the practice alive. Now, I'm selective as to whose regime I try to change and I don't have those conversations with patients every day like before.

I'm disappointed with my job. I get angry. Sometimes, it makes me irritable. I have to catch myself because that's not who I am. I am a nurturer at heart. I'm kind, I care probably way too much. I worked so hard to get to where I'm at and I enjoy what I do, minus the opioids, [*Laugh*] There's good and bad with everything. There's not going to be a perfect job where you're going to like everything all the time.

I fear that I may become more cynical in future years; I find glimpses of that now. When I have a new patient, I already judge them before I walk in the door. I look at their paperwork and pharmacy board and automatically put them in a box. I know what they're going to say and I'm right 80% of the time. It disturbs me because I don't want to be that judgmental person.

I can't see how to change things without stopping being a pain physician. [*Laugh*] I've thought, "Maybe I don't belong here." I mean, if I don't see much pathology on MRI and they haven't tried conservative therapies, if their pain scores are an eight out of ten and they are on high-dose opioids, I feel we need to reduce and see if they have opioid hyperalgesia or something else that is contributing to their pain. Whereas, my colleagues just do the status quo, "Let's just refill, let's just make them happy, that's what they want anyway."

I feel that medicine has changed drastically over time. The pharmaceutical companies and the government are dictating what we do. Medicare guidelines look at patients' satisfaction scores. In a pain clinic, the outcome should be how much we reduce opioids, how many people we treat who are pain-free without them. We need to reward pain clinics that use less resources, that are more cost-effective and efficient at treating pain, rather than just putting on a sticking plaster, like giving an opioid.

Sometimes there are threatening situations. I am petite and Hispanic and patients think I'm younger than I am. Both male and female patients, once I challenge them to reduce their opioids a little, will ask me, "Have you ever been in pain? I think you should feel pain." Or they'll use abusive language toward me and walk out the door, making me feel bad for not giving them what they wanted. I've had to go to my office to cry and not have my staff see me in that vulnerable position. Other times, the abuse happens right in front of my staff.

But there's nothing for me to feel bad about at the end of the day. That behavior is not my problem. But it feels humiliating. It's disrespectful.

Sometimes, I've had to have a medical assistant in the room in case things get too heated. At one point, I had a patient, saying, "Well, I understand where you are coming from, I know you can't refill my prescription because...." They'd tested positive for illegal drugs. They lifted their padded coat and there was a gun!

Another patient who tested positive for illegal drugs was told over the phone that we were going to terminate the opioid agreement. He said, "I'm going to go down there myself and tell you in person how I really feel." At that point, we had to alert the police because that's a threat. This is not the way I thought I was going to practice medicine, where I would be afraid of what my patients would do in retaliation.

I vent almost daily to my colleagues, and to my friends. [*Laugh*] I have learned to use humor in my practice. That's the only thing that's keeping me going, and just knowing that at some point, the patient will be open to change. It's not what I thought I'd signed up for when I started out as a medical student. Absolutely not. [*Sighs*] I didn't think it was going to be this stressful. [*Laugh*] I'm spiritual and I'm hoping that there is a practice that either I can start or join that is more aligned with my ideals, my ethics. I don't want to stop helping people.

I just feel sad. I'm the first of my family to graduate from college, and then from medical school. [*Tearfully*] I know my parents are really proud of me and I just don't want to walk away. I've thought about going into another field of medicine, maybe dermatology. [*Laugh*] You don't see any violent people there, I would imagine! [*Laugh*] But it would take a lot of time to apply, go through residency and then get board certified. I've wanted to be a doctor since the age of ten, so there's no way that I'm going to stop!

## Discussion or Writing Prompts

1 Dr Heredia describes feeling despair over being pressured to practice medicine in a manner that she had not expected. "Moral injury" results when one feels powerless against the complicity demanded by a system that goes against one's ethical values. Recall a time

when you encountered a feeling of "moral injury." How did you recognize and respond to it? Assess alternative responses.

2  Discuss a time when something was harder than expected and describe how you navigated the situation.

3  "I usually give in because I see that they're suffering. I feel their resistance to change and their fear." Describe a situation where you "gave in" due to not wanting a person to suffer, even though you didn't think it was right.

4  What is the difference between patient satisfaction and meeting the needs of the patient? How can we guard against compromising the needs of the patient to get a good patient satisfaction score?

5  "There's not going to be a perfect job where you're going to like everything all the time." What allows you to cope with the things you don't like in your job?

6  "When I have a new patient, I already judge them before I walk in the door." Think of a time when you judged a patient's character or diagnosis without talking with them. Even if your snap judgment seemed correct, what did you lose by making it? How do you identify and manage feelings of cynicism concerning patients?

7  Describe a situation in which you were able to channel your anger for good.

8  Recall a time when you faced a loss of physical or psychological safety at work and how that situation was, or should have been, addressed.

# Part VIII
# Addiction

# 25 Road to Recovery

*Dr Phil Lincoln was addicted to drugs and alcohol in college and throughout his residency training. In the years leading up to sobriety, he could not picture an existence without them. He firmly believed he needed substances to have fun, to relax, to quiet his thoughts and cope with life's challenges. Giving up substances completely seemed impossible. It turns out that his life in recovery is far better than he ever imagined it could be.*

I grew up in a family fractured by a long history of alcoholism. My mother was raised in a chaotic household by her alcoholic mother and my father's father was an abusive, violent alcoholic who ultimately died by suicide while my father, also a physician, was in medical school. My parents divorced when I was around five years old, and they have each been through at least five divorces, so I got used to taking care of myself and supporting my mom. I spent a lot of time with my mother's family because my father worked far away. My mom's brother had a closed head injury when he was in college because of drinking and driving, and he lived with my grandparents who cared for him, so I saw a lot of consequences of drinking, but I didn't understand what it all meant. I was certain though that I was not going to drink and expose myself to those risks.

Fast forward to high school. I was achieving very well academically but I was not particularly happy from a social perspective; I wanted to have more friends, to fit in and enjoy life. I started drinking and shortly after that started using drugs, pharmaceutical and hallucinogenic, and that continued through college and became a central part of my social life. Drinking and doing drugs in high school was a lot of fun. I met new people and we went to concerts and parties, but I always had this feeling in the back of my head that what I was doing was dangerous. I stayed away from the hard stuff because I was a little bit worried about what might happen.

Throughout high school and college I was very dedicated to my studies and once I had an accomplishment, I rewarded myself with drink and drugs. If my grades dropped in any way, I would attempt to control my drinking, pulling back and recalibrating. There is something called Antabuse (disulfiram) and I had friends who were court-ordered to take it because they drank and

DOI: 10.4324/9781003475170-33

got DUIs. But they took it and still abused; some of them drank past it; some would take other drugs to negate its effects. I thought about taking it to control my abusing, but I didn't use it. Instead, I got very involved in extracurricular activities that required me not to drink and I was even involved in an organization that made me sign a pledge not to do drugs. I made that commitment but broke it immediately because drugs and drink were such a part of my life at that point that I couldn't resist.

I became more compulsive about this cycle when I went through medical school. I was constantly in a state of both rationalization and frustration. I studied very hard, did very well, far better than in college, all A's, top of my class. I would work then binge; a very regular cycle. At that point, I felt very in control of my usage, because I was highly motivated to do well in medical school. And at the point that I got to residency, I married a young lady I'd met in college. She was very permissive, but also a very nice person and I felt committed to doing right by her.

After our marriage, I had probably my longest period of abstinence, about three months. And throughout my internship, I didn't drink, but I smoked a lot of pot. Then I got to residency and I restarted my cycle. I was using drugs and drinking but felt like I was still doing well and achieving, and I eventually started relaxing my control. I began giving myself permission to drink and use more drugs because there were no tests and I was getting good evaluations in my residency.

I wanted to end every day intoxicated in some way, feeling the relief of drugs or alcohol. With drink it was never the taste I was after; it was the effect. While normal people may want to go home and have a glass of wine, that's never how it's been for me. If I had a glass of wine, it meant that I was drinking the bottle. Putting a limit on myself was not something that I wanted anymore. So as I neared the end of my residency, I asked for a divorce from my wife so I could continue to drink and use drugs freely. She didn't know I was abusing because I was hiding it from her; I would do everything out of sight, in the garage or the basement. I decided it was better for me to stop lying and to end the relationship. That was how distorted my thinking was. I feel terrible about all that now and I never want to have to hide things again like that.

After the divorce, I spent the next year drinking and doing drugs, almost without limit. I was beginning to dangerously use in circumstances when I would be on call, or when I was going to go in later in the day. Again, I never had any consequences in my job; my evaluations said that I was a competent and hardworking resident so, from my perspective, my work never suffered. However, my relationships with the people I worked with suffered dramatically. I was angry and hostile, unpleasant to be around. My co-residents and my faculty were afraid of me because of my attitude, and I was very resentful about everything. My life was a disaster.

My addiction was a feedback loop, and I carried a lot of anger from the way my life had become. My interaction with the world was rooted in resentment and righteous indignation, and on top of that, I felt guilt and shame and remorse about the way I was behaving. But I only knew how to manage those emotions by pouring in more drugs and alcohol.

The effect it could have on my career was my biggest worry. Throughout my entire adult life, from the point of high school through my residency, I was terrified. I feared that I would be like my dad, who struggled through his own career problems due to anger issues. I feared that something would happen and I would lose my job, and everything I had worked so hard to achieve would be taken from me.

A simple drug test would have revealed what I was doing. Along the way, I had been pulled over numerous times while intoxicated or under the influence with illegal substances on me. I'd had my car searched but never experienced a consequence, and that is inexplicable to me. I didn't see how unmanageable my life was. It didn't matter that I was lucky to have run out of gas on the side of the road because I was so drunk that otherwise I probably would've wrecked my car in the 40-mile drive home from the bar. I was never held to account, but that prevented me from getting the help that I needed for a really long time.

Then I got into another relationship and this person was more willing to tell me what my issues were. I began to hear some feedback that I had a drinking problem, which I knew I did but thought that I was managing. Even when I'd put myself in positions where I could have been violently injured, I always thought I was different, that I was better than other people, that I wouldn't be affected the way they were.

What happened was that the woman I was seeing went away for New Year's Eve and I told her, "I'm going to go to a block party. It's gonna be families and friends in my neighborhood. I'm not gonna go downtown Madison to have a wild time." I subsequently got really, really intoxicated at the event and did some regrettable things that severely embarrassed me. Some of the people in attendance showed up at my house a day later and said, "We need to know that you're going to get help because the way that you act and behave is unacceptable. If you don't get help, then we're going to notify the people you work with that you have a problem." And they openly asked me, "Do you have an explanation for this?" And I said, "I think I have a drinking problem."

That was the first time I'd admitted it to people. And those neighbors and friends changed my life.

I told my new partner what had happened, and she was supportive, but ultimately that relationship didn't survive. There were a lot of big changes that I had to make to myself, and I think both of us realized that we were not prepared to go through it all together.

When I got that ultimatum from those neighbors and friends, I felt the bottom dropping out of my life. This was the moment that I had been dreading and I could fall or I could make a step in the right direction. I'd said I would get some help, but I did not know what that meant, so I went back and sat on my couch and did drugs again. A couple of days later, I did drugs for the last time. I knew it was time to stop.

We had a residency support program at my hospital, and I made an appointment with the psychiatrist. I was absolutely terrified about any consequences, but I was willing to accept that risk because I knew the way I was going would lead to something far worse. It had been clear to me, standing on my front porch talking to those people, that my disastrous behavior was going to accelerate.

I told my story to the psychiatrist, and she said I should try an outpatient treatment program. She assured me that there would be no consequences and that everything would be fine. I trusted her because I didn't know what else to do.

So, I went to the intensive outpatient program that was offered through my hospital system. I let my program director know what was going on and she was extremely supportive. She made sure that I had the time I needed because my therapy group met for two months immediately after work, so I had to leave about 30 minutes early. I told people that I had a doctor's appointment, and only once did I get pushback, and I simply referred that individual to my program director. I completed the program, and it was the hardest couple of months that I had been through in terms of not using and not drinking. I was confronting a lot of things, and I was scared and still not feeling 100% better when it ended.

It was the time we were starting to study for our boards, and I went to meet my psychologist who was reviewing me at post-treatment. I was feeling really angry. I'd had a bad encounter with one of my faculty during a board review and my frustration had flared. I didn't drink over it, but I was in a negative headspace about everything. And my psychologist asked me one question, "Have you been doing anything else since you finished the treatment?" And I said, "No, I did the program. I'm not drinking. I'm okay." He's like, "Do you feel okay?" and I said, "No." He said, "You should try something else; you should go and talk to people." So I went to my first Caduceus group meeting, which is a recovery group for healthcare providers. That was the first "safe space" I walked into.

It was a strange, unusual experience. We said the serenity prayer and I didn't know the language and couldn't see the point of it. We talked a lot about ourselves, about things I was not comfortable talking about, and I listened, but it was giving me insight into my problems. I went back again, and I met some physicians who extended their hands to me and gave me their phone numbers and I called them because I had found this kernel of willingness to take help. And that grew and I started connecting with people.

Then later, I went to my first true Alcoholics Anonymous meeting in the outside community which was more rooted in how to solve the problems on a daily basis. It was so hard for me to go that first time. There were hundreds of people in the room. Hundreds! I was afraid of seeing people who might know me, afraid they'd recognize me or would intuitively know that I was a doctor.

I remember walking out of that meeting and meeting with some of my friends who did not have problems with drugs and alcohol, and they asked me how long I would have to keep going there. I said, "I don't know," and then I cried. That was almost 12 years ago.

As to my work, I never had a lapse in my training when getting my credentials for fellowship. I was required to sign up for a monitoring program and submit to drug tests and counseling because I disclosed that I had gone through treatment. That felt hard because it was a consequence of being honest. But it was also a gift; it gave me the space to continue working on my recovery knowing that there was a safety net beneath me and knowing that there were people looking out for me. I completed my monitoring—it was not really a major problem—and I've never had difficulty getting a job or when I've disclosed information to other people. In my current work, when I shared my situation with my future Chair, she said it was an asset, and she was glad to know that about me.

I know I've been granted a daily reprieve from drinking or doing drugs by virtue of my commitment to my recovery. I don't have to get intoxicated to cope with life. I discovered that there is a lot of life to be lived so I became very active. I ran a marathon in my first year of sobriety; I trained for a triathlon and competed in that, and then I got very involved in academics. I started working harder on career things that I was already interested in, and the time fills up because you build more relationships with people.

I met my present partner when I was six months into recovery, so she has never known me to drink or use drugs and she has supported me and shown me a lot about myself. I have learned to be willing to work on myself, to be patient and tolerant and honest and open-minded and accepting of my imperfections and those of others. Those things didn't come easily to me because I wasn't used to accepting anything short of excellence.

Now my partner and I have a young child and my continuing commitment to my sobriety is also for my family. I know that there are genetic predispositions to addiction, but I have learnt in recovery that there are things I cannot allow myself to be afraid of.

I also have very close relationships with my mom and dad and other members of my family. Due to my recovery process, the depth of our relationships has really increased. We have incredible conversations because of our mutual understanding about what I went through and how it relates to what they experienced in their lives.

If you go to Alcoholics Anonymous, you have a sponsor who supports and helps you through the 12 steps of the program, and in doing that, you develop a relationship. Your sponsor is always another person in recovery. Mine now has a completely different job than me and he's 15 years older. I found him after I moved cities when I stood up at an AA meeting and said, I need a sponsor. I need someone to work with me and take me through the steps again. And a man came up to me after the meeting and we've been working together since. He told me, "I want you to call me every day." And I, a physician with 11 years of sobriety, didn't say anything. I was like, "Okay." And so I do call him all the time, and it helps me stay in the mindset of asking for help.

His own sponsor has fewer years of sobriety than him, but he's very dedicated to the program. We get together on Sunday morning. It's an informal meeting: me, my sponsor, and my sponsor's sponsor, a group of men all connected in their recovery. We share what's going on and how our recovery relates to our life experiences. It gives a feeling of connectedness that you don't get in other places, and the only way I could have found that was through seeking help. It is a gift.

The program of recovery offered through the AA 12 steps is one that relies on the concept of a higher power, and anyone can come into the program and define their higher power as what they want it to be. If you want, you can call it God, and they do use the term God. A friend says that when we talk about God and our higher power, we consider it a term of art. It is something we use as a reference point when we are turning ourselves over to something other than ourselves. Some people say it can be like an engine block that sits in your living room; it does not have to be something in the heavens. So, I go back to where I came from, which was an agnostic/atheist, and I have a really tough time accepting that there is some grand plan in the universe when things are very challenging. But I do know that when there is no one else for me to ask for help, when I just need to talk to somebody, I turn to the higher power. I don't know who that is or if they'll answer. But I know that I'm not the person I need to talk to about solving my problems.

Today I am perfectly fine being around people drinking. I have times when, if there is a great deal of intoxication or things are wild, I may need to step away; I have learned when it is the right time for me to leave. We have alcohol in our home and it's not a problem; I would never drink again. There is no other way for me to live but in a substance-free life because my instinct is still to want to change the way I feel by using something external.

If other physicians feel they have a problem with addiction, I'd say don't be scared to ask for help or to talk to someone about it. Do not be afraid to be flawed or imperfect. Do not be afraid of the consequences of seeking help. And importantly, know you're not alone. I have friends connected through recovery and we talk regularly. I attend meetings, I work with others outside of my own career and I'm constantly trying to find ways to help. I'm so personally grateful that someone helped me, saved me.

I know I am more receptive to the struggles of others than I ever was before, and I strive to be a better colleague and friend and physician. The ability to connect with people is extremely important to me because I felt so disconnected for so long. I'm even a wellness leader for my department at my hospital and my relationship with my colleagues is wonderful! Which comes a great surprise to my old friends who thought of me as the grouchiest individual around. So, life has all worked out and it's better than I ever imagined it could be. I'm very happy!

**Discussion or Writing Prompts**

1  Dr Lincoln was determined not to follow in a family member's footsteps, but that didn't protect him from developing addiction. Describe your experiences in trying to overcome a barrier to a positive lifestyle, e.g., substances, food, sedentary lifestyle.
2  "I felt guilt and shame and remorse about the way I was behaving. But I only knew how to manage those emotions by pouring in more drugs and alcohol." Discuss a feedback loop of emotions and behaviors that dug you deeper.
3  The threat that Dr Lincoln's friends might notify his workplace about his drinking helped motivate him to seek help. Recall a time when confronting a friend about their behavior or hidden condition was what they needed.
4  Despite its intrusiveness, Dr Lincoln found that the monitoring program he had to sign up for (often called Physician Health Program (PHP)) was a positive support and safety net rather than a barrier in his career. Explore how PHPs are perceived and how they can indeed help physicians.
5  "In my current work, when I shared my situation with my future Chair, she said it was an asset, and she was glad to know that about me." Discuss the role of leadership and organizational support in reducing stigma and aiding engagement in recovery.
6  Dr Lincoln stresses that a key factor in his recovery is being willing to ask for help rather than trying to solve all his problems alone. Think about a time that you struggled to ask for help. What made it difficult? What can be done to make it easier to seek help?

## Resources

International Doctors in Alcoholics Anonymous. (n.d.). https://www.idaa.org/.
  Alcoholics Anonymous. (n.d.). https://www.aa.org/.
  National Institute on Alcohol Abuse and Alcoholism. (n.d.). https://alcoholtreatment.niaaa.nih.gov/.

# 26 Practicing Medicine in the Grasp of Addiction

*Dr Barry Benson has recently retired from a long career owning and running health care facilities. His account of his spiral into addiction and then recovery is startlingly honest. Along the way, he provides useful information about programs for children of physicians affected by addiction.*

## Part 1. Spiral into Addiction

I think the underpinnings of my addiction probably go all the way back to childhood experiences. I grew up in a family where my father was a heavy drinker. He may have been an alcoholic, but he never admitted to himself that there was a real problem. He manipulated things to the point where he could continue without getting in trouble. And he was very overwhelming in terms of his need to control. So, all his children had to become professionals.

Later in life he got confronted by the family. My mom was seeing a psychiatrist, and the family met with the psychiatrist and invited my dad along. And everybody said to him, "We're worried about you. It seems like your drinking is progressing. You know you're having fights with Mom." He said, "I don't have a problem with drinking; I'll show you. I'll never drink whiskey again." And then he started drinking beer in excess. [*Laugh*] So that was his solution to his quote, "drinking problem."

I guess smoking was my first drug and I snuck cigarettes when I was 10, 11, 12 years old. I felt this thrill about getting away with it. I was a child of the sixties and coming of age in that era was pretty radical, the Beatles and the Vietnam War and all that stuff. We didn't trust anybody over 30; the older generation was clueless; we were just gonna do what felt good; free love, sex, drugs, rock and roll, and we're gonna be changing the world. Yeah, that was '67! I was a hippy in college and that's when my drug use started, when LSD was still legal.

I was an undergraduate and my friends were being sent to Vietnam. We were protesting and burning our draft cards and escaping to Canada. To me drugs were everywhere and everyone was doing it, but looking back, I can see that the people who were doing it congregated together.

DOI: 10.4324/9781003475170-34

To be a successful student at my university you had to maintain a semblance of sanity; it was full of really smart people. My drugs and alcohol use started to escalate there because I was very shy, terrible at interacting with people except when I met the friends who were smoking pot, doing drugs, and then we had this instant bond. My standard was that it didn't matter how many drugs I was using provided I did well in college, because success to my parents was good grades. My dad was like, "You're going be a doctor," and I had to follow his rules, be good in school.

In college, I was in two crowds: the very intellectual, educated crowd, and then back home was the hippie crowd, the drug crowd. So I hung out with the bad people on the weekends and good people during the week. Then I got introduced to even harder drugs, when my druggie friends were starting with cocaine and even snorting heroin, and some guys got into injecting it, but I never injected.

I just kept the things separate, and I was able to escalate the drug use and not bottom out in classes, and my dad was happy. But I did find those drug weekends were something I yearned for.

There was a lot of LSD and pills around my college town so we'd invite our friends up for the weekend and just blitz out, and then Monday morning it was time to go to work. So, Friday night started the weekend and Sunday night was off limits, until it wasn't. Then, gradually, it began on Thursday and went till Sunday night and you woke up Monday and needed something to get through the day. The timeframe of the drug-taking expanded, but I had to maintain this aura of being fine.

I was a psych major and as a senior, I was a teaching fellow in the Psych 101 class. I taught a group of 10 or 12 students and we studied the psychology of drugs. I knew everything about it! Our final exam was a drug party at my house, and the professor came because he was very tolerant, and we had a punchbowl and people would just throw in pills. Nobody knew what was in there and everyone would take what they wanted. We had a tank of nitrous oxide too. And the professor, we had to lift him off the couch and drop him off at his front door. It was all kind of acceptable behavior, wild!

Psychology interested me because I had been abused sexually by my brother as a young child, so there was this black hole in my soul, something wrong within, and that made me timid and afraid that people would find out and walk away thinking I was tainted. The drugs were my escape from myself, you know. But I was just lonely inside, even in a crowd.

At medical school it was hard to find people like me. Out of, maybe, 200 people in my class, there was only a group of 10 or 15 that drank a lot and went to hockey games with cases of beer.

I was a medical school hippie. The hippies were at the fringe of the class, smoking pot and partying a lot. Most of the students were just deadly serious. They were scientists. Some of 'em were going to medical school just to be able to do research. They already had their careers planned out, whereas I had no clue. I was just kind of drifting along, but I was still able to do everything I had to do.

I was educated beyond my intelligence. I just had a great memory; I was a perfect test taker. No matter what I'd been doing, I could always give myself a week to go over the material and take notes and learn everything I needed and spit it back out, because the only thing that mattered were the scores. So every two weeks I'd get engaged deeply in the study, and then afterward it was celebration time, and I'd go on a bender for a few days.

I was kind of afraid of being a doctor. It was too much responsibility for me. It was life and death stuff, and I was like, "I don't know if I can do that." I couldn't select a career, so I drifted through different things. The first one was psychiatry. Psychology as an undergrad and psychiatry as a medical student was a way of dealing with the deep dark inside me without having to ask for help. I thought if I'd learn enough, I'd self-administer the treatment. Crazy! [*Laugh*] But the drugs and alcohol were accelerating as the way to combat my fears.

Drugs and alcohol study was just neglected at medical school. We only spent five days studying them. And when you were treating patients back then, everybody with an obvious drug or alcohol issue was deemed to be deficient in their ability to make the right choices. They knew right from wrong but were choosing wrong because they were drug addicts and alcoholics, so they were treated with disdain and always put in the room at the end of the hall. And the rounds with the professors always ended up with, "I'm gonna discharge you and tell you that if you don't stop, you're gonna die," and then they were back a month later and the professor is treating these people as if they were mentally negligent or as if they had the capacity to choose the right thing. Alcoholism was not considered a disease; it was treated like a moral deficiency.

At medical school, toward the end, I was just hanging on. And in the last year you were no longer under the microscope; all you had to do was pass the forerunner of the USMLE exams. If you got past the first, you're good. And then you do Part 2; you pass that, you're good. Those were the only markers. And obviously I was able to do those things because of my excellent memory.

But my clinical stuff was very weak. I wasn't well prepared for rounds and being grilled by the attending. My knowledge base wasn't sufficient when I had mystery patients and was told to go and do the half-hour assessment and then explain what was wrong with the person. I had no clue really; I had to be prepped by the resident. There was a one-year-old with severe anemia in pediatrics, and you're supposed to know the basics, but I didn't. I wasn't prepared 'cause I neglected studies where I wasn't forced to learn for exams. You were supposed to learn the clinical stuff on your own, but I was too "out there" to do that. I wasn't even sure what I wanted to do.

I finally ended up applying for some surgery residencies because that instantaneous gratification of seeing somebody being really sick one day and really better the next day just thrilled me. I didn't even think about how dangerous surgery could be. I didn't think about having somebody's life and death in my hands. And then, you know, reality struck. My first patient died, and I couldn't get over the fact that I'd said he could go take a shower after his MI (heart attack). But he had such a weakened cardiac left ventricle that it burst and he died, so I was responsible. I was poorly trained. I knew I'd missed the relevant day in class.

And I'm moonlighting in the ERs and I had a drunk patient come in who had suffered a head injury. He was unconscious and then woke up somewhat disoriented. There was no cat scan imaging in those days, so I called the neurosurgery chief resident. I said, "Look, I've got a guy with a head injury, I think he needs to have an angiogram." That was the only way you could do a brain anatomy. And he says, "You know, it's midnight. Are you sure? I don't wanna have to come in there." I said, "Okay." And then the guy died the next morning of a subdural hematoma. It could have been evacuated; he could've lived. I got called down to the pathology autopsy to be shown what I had done wrong. These things created my fear that I wouldn't make it in this field. And then all these people are coming in with these lame suicide attempts, and I'm just getting mad. I said, "If you wanna do a suicide, you might as well do it right. I should write you a manual so you don't just come in here with your wrist slit in the wrong spot."

And then I had a woman with postpartum depression within like a week or two of delivery, and she just took a gun up to her left chest and shot herself. She just missed her heart, but she hit a small pulmonary vein. Initially she appeared stable, but we took an X-ray and there was obviously a large amount of blood that had collected in her chest. A true surgeon would have said, "Get a chest tube. We have to evacuate this immediately," but I just ended up calling the chief resident who was in charge of the ER that night and he came and said, "What's wrong with you? Why didn't you use the chest tube? Don't you know how?" And then I just kept backing away further.

When I finally met a hand surgeon, I saw that his was the safest kind of surgery—he called it "gentleman surgery." You put this guy on the table, put an Esmarch dressing on his arm so there's no blood flow, put on a cuff to cut off the circulation and the arm looks like a cadaver's. So, we're sitting with this arm out to the side on the hand table and we're looking through the microscope and doing arteries and nerves and veins. But if we screw it up, he'd only lose the finger, not like life and death stuff. So that became my next idea. I was gonna do hand surgery, but I couldn't do that without finishing the surgery residency first.

At that point I was using more narcotics and working 72-hour shifts. When you're a surgeon, you just stayed there because all you wanted to do was more operations to get trained. It was 120 hours a week in-house. When I had a day off, I just went home and got high the whole time. I stole and collected drugs because I'd moved to the northwest for residency training and my friends who got me drugs were gone. The drugs were the only thing that calmed me down enough to face the world.

## Part 2.  Consequences

I'd started writing prescriptions; pretending they were for my aunt, my uncle, my sister, my brother. I would go to the pharmacy and pretend that I was Uncle Joe and this doctor had given me the prescription and then I'd take and use the drugs. I was caught because I worried that one day they'd see all these prescriptions I'm writing and decide to investigate, so I started using other doctors' names to sign the prescriptions. And then the inevitable happened. I was using a university pad and probably wrote out an excessive amount of narcotics and unbeknownst to me, the pharmacy called the house. When I walked out the door with the bottle of pills the cops were waiting for me. They had called the hospital and found that the doctor did not write that prescription and there was no patient by that name and I'd just made it all up. I got handcuffed and fingerprinted and they took the two pictures with the number on your chest and I went to jail. I had a lawyer cousin who got me bailed out the next morning.

At that point I was married and our first child had been born, and my drug use escalated because I was incapable of supporting her and my wife. I knew I was going to fail at surgery and I was terrified. I was teaching residents and interns and we'd be up at midnight doing things like a serious appendix rupture. I was the third-year resident so I was the one trained, and I'd be feeling like, "Is this person gonna die?" I used to be able to talk to the senior resident who would help me through this, but now we're alone at midnight with a kid. I was just terrified. I was just overwhelmed.

The day after I was arrested, having to face the Medical Board loomed in my mind and I raced to the conclusion that it was all over. "You're gonna lose your license. Nobody else is going to let you be a doctor." I had this kid that's eight weeks old and I'd purchased a million-dollar life insurance policy, and if your death was accidental, it doubled. I figure, "Okay, I'm worthless. I'll never be able to show my head again. If I only could die accidentally, that would solve everything."

We lived near lots of beautiful mountains and valleys and rivers. I knew everywhere in the vicinity and chose a place with rocky cliffs with scenic highways along the edge. The cliffs go down about 900 feet. With my disdain at suicide victims who it fucked it up, I said, "Well, if I accidentally have a car go over this cliff, then there's no way I could possibly survive 900 feet."

On the way to driving out there, my wife said, "Why are you up at five in the morning?" I made up a stupid reason like we're out of bread. But I had the plan; it seemed like a perfect solution. I'd had some alcohol and bought antifreeze because I was worried that if I couldn't go through with driving over the cliff, at least I'd die from the antifreeze poisoning.

Antifreeze comes in gallon size and I'm drinking it and driving and crying and being like in a different world, terrified of not being able to do this. Then

I found the perfect spot. I backed up the car and drove off. The car careened and that was the last thing I remember. It turned out the car had struck a tree about 80 feet over the edge as it came crashing down that 900-foot drop. There was an article in the paper quoting the firemen that pulled the hulk of the car out, and he said the rear bumper was resting against a sapling. That was the only thing preventing the car from going all the way down.

I woke up late afternoon, blood everywhere, the windows blown out and the car kind of crushed, so I'd obviously failed: I was alive. I'd broken three vertebrae; the bones were crushed, there was compression, but it wasn't a spine spinal cord injury. So now I'm in this car and I said, "Maybe if I just scrape off all these scabs, I'll bleed to death." And then I was out again, probably from the head injury and probably from the poisoning. Turns out alcohol is the treatment for antifreeze poisoning; I forgot that day. I guess I wasn't thinking straight, [*Laugh*] but, yeah, alcohol is the treatment, so I was pretreated—the antifreeze didn't kill me!

I woke up and tore the scabs off and it was dusk and I'm hearing the sounds of birds. I'm on the side of a cliff and you can't see the car from the road. It's only really used by tourists on the weekend mostly. And, you know, the birds are gonna pluck out my eyeballs! I'd read a book about birds plucking eyeballs so I had to get outta there. I somehow crawled from this crushed vehicle and slowly pulled myself up to the road and I still remember grabbing roots and branches and finding a foothold. I want to be dead, but I don't wanna be awake and die slowly by being devoured by rodents. So eventually I did make it to the road and luckily somebody at night was using this highway. I remember the car pulling over and they said, "Oh my God, what happened to you?" I said, "My car accidentally, you know ...." And so I ended up at my own hospital.

I'd already decided that I couldn't do the next year, the fourth year. I was gonna take a year off and I'd organized a Michigan license, and I'd interviewed for jobs there. I thought, "Well, I know ER stuff, that'll be safe. That's not as scary; you can either treat them or admit them to somebody else; you're not really the person responsible." In my head, ER would be a more controlled environment where there would be somebody around if I needed help. So I got a job and found a place to live and I was gonna start in July. And it was June the eighth when I got arrested.

So obviously the job didn't work out. [*Laugh*] I had faced the Board after my accident, and they didn't jerk my license but restricted it for ten years. I wasn't to write narcotic prescriptions and I had to see a psychiatrist. My brain was so traumatized from the head injury that it's been permanently affected. In the MRI of my brain, there's an absent spot in the right frontal lobe. It's all white and it should be gray. It's all scar tissue.

I didn't get referred for treatment of my addiction after almost killing myself, for being busted for illegal use of drugs. I got sent to a shrink for suicidal physicians. They just diagnosed me completely incorrectly.

So then I called my new boss in Michigan. I said, "There's been a little glitch." She said, "Don't even bother." But I didn't have a residency slot 'cause I'd already elected not to take one the next year, so we just ended up moving anyway.

I had this broken back and was getting lots of free narcotics. Legitimate. [*Laugh*] That kind of took the place of having illegally obtained stuff! I had my Michigan license and I self-reported there. They didn't have communication between medical boards at that point, so I could have gone to Michigan and just lied, but I figured I'd better let them know, and they restricted me for just one year.

But I couldn't find work because I couldn't prescribe so I ended up working in a plasmapheresis center; that's where down-and-outs come. They have a liter of blood drawn and instead of donating whole blood, the plasma is retained. They give the guy 20 bucks and reinfuse their blood cells so they can come back every two weeks and get 20 bucks.

Meanwhile, I had a metal frame to keep my spine straight. It kept me from bending, twisting, or leaning. I had to wear that all day and take it off in bed at night. So I'm sitting in this office wearing this metal cage and a white coat on top and a tie and then come these patients. No prescriptions, no treatment. I had to like say, "He's okay to donate today," or whatever. And that was my first "prestigious" medical job. [*Laugh*]

I just lied to my wife. I told her I'd had an accident, and then the arrest had come up and I pretended they were separate. I know she knew they weren't but we never really discussed it. Incredible denial. And we did everything together. We smoked cigarettes, used drugs, but the day she found out she was pregnant, I said we're stopping everything. Like cold Turkey, no smoking, drinking, drugs. I'd been in obstetrics!

She stopped but I couldn't. That's the difference between an addict and a heavy user. A heavy user, given a sufficient reason, can stop or moderate but an addict cannot. I tried to stop; it didn't work, then I said I'd taper off. But I started lying, pretending I was on call. I'd be in some motel with a legal prescription bottle full of pills, not thinking I had an addiction because I wasn't using every day and didn't have withdrawal.

I worked at the plasma place for six months and then I found a clinic doing industrial medicine, like workers' injury. A physician working in the industrial medicine clinic felt sorry for me and I was brought in to do sales. My dad had a business and he'd told me that no matter what you do in life, if you know how to sell, it'll enhance your career. So I started getting engaged in the sales and I learned the business from the partner. And then they said, we're gonna build more places. We want you to join us, so I became a junior partner. And then it became wildly successful, beyond my imagination.

I'd worked with this hand surgeon and had learned enough so that when a patient came in with hand injuries, I could treat them and not have to refer them, so I became even more useful. We kept expanding, and we ended up owning 14 clinics. But I was stealing drugs from my own clinic. And then the senior partner said, "I wanna retire and I want all my money right now." So they sold these clinics for $14 million in 1985 and I got 10% of it. I'd worked there for six years. Crazy!

I knew my record was so bleak that I could never get a real job. That was gonna be it. But the partners who'd bought the business were interested in a subspecialty called occupational medicine and wanted me to stay. I thought, "Well, I have enough money to retire now," and they said, "We'll pay you triple what you used to make and we'll give you 5% of the ownership every year you stay with us." It was crazy, remarkable!

I bought the fancy house with a swimming pool and hot tub and the fancy cars, and the two kids were taken care of and everything looked good. It proved to everyone, including myself that I didn't have a problem.

Then another hospital offered to build a clinic if I would manage and direct it, and I didn't have to put any money into it, so I did that. It was just another gift being thrown my way. But I was still drinking and using drugs illegally, but not getting in trouble. Getting caught was my real worry. Every day I woke I would say, "I'm a fake, I'm a pretense. I'm not a real doctor. I'm a liar, cheater, stealer, living like I deserve all these gifts, and I don't."

Meanwhile, there was a lot of turmoil at home. I'd show up for things like a dance recital, either recovering from my last drinking or drugging, or sit in the audience looking at my watch, waiting to escape and get drunk, or I was high. Those were the only three states. In occupational medicine, they called it the disease of presenteeism, that's when you're physically there, but not functioning as you should be. You're locked in the future or past, not in the moment. You're physically present, but not functioning.

I thought I didn't have a problem because I was getting away with it all. [*Laugh*] I was using drugs with my cousin Billy who grew up with us. Billy was milking drugs from doctors; that was before they charted who's prescribing what to whom. He had five different doctors he'd go to at various times for his drugs and I was getting samples from the big pharma. Whenever he got drugs he'd split them with me and whenever I got samples, I'd split 'em with him and we would use together. Then he got to the point where he decided he had a problem and sought help from my older brother who was a doctor, and Billy ended up going to treatment.

There he learned all about the 12-step Alcoholics Anonymous program. The first step is admission and then you're supposed to go through the whole process until you have a message to carry to a new person needing help. Billy was enthralled with giving back and helping others so he said to my brother, "If you think I'm bad, your own brother's way worse." So that's when I got diagnosed.

## Part 3. Recovery

My brother was a really good doctor with a family practice, and I'd long forgiven him for the sexual assault from when we were children. He knew from Billy what was going on. Then he saw some things about my behavior that were concerning, like falling asleep at the basketball game or nodding off in the car. He knew exactly what was going on, but I wasn't ready to hear it. I knew I was lying, cheating, stealing, and doing, but I was getting away with it, so in my mind, there was no real problem. I could not see the truth right in front of my eyes.

I was just like the guy in that back ward when I was training, with the yellow jaundice and bleeding out of the esophagus. And then when you're ready to discharge the person you say, "Look, you just about died, can't you see how bad this drinking thing is?" And they come back a month later, and you say, "You idiot. How could you possibly have gone and done this again? Can't you see what's wrong with you?" And that was my same thing.

My brother understood the disease and, and he says, "You and Billy are the same. Why don't you seek help?" I was pretty much ready to agree that all was not going swimmingly, so I thought "I'll try it." I ended up going for a four-day evaluation, and I didn't really think I was that bad. But it didn't take 'em four days to figure out that I really needed inpatient treatment.

Meanwhile I'd gotten in a fight with the main partner of the place that had enticed me to help set up the clinics and he fired me: "We're gonna let you go into some distant clinic out in the boondocks. Or you have 12 weeks' notice and you could leave today." That freed my schedule up to allow me to go to a treatment center designed for healthcare professionals.

The treatment center is deeply oriented toward the 12-step AA program. All the state boards would send their sick doctors there because they wanted to guarantee they got long-term treatment, because the smarter you are, the more resistant you are to seeing the truth. I went there because my brother's friend went to the same treatment center and his friend was worse than me, but with a story very similar to mine. The thoughts, feelings, and behaviors, all that stuff that's different about alcoholics or addicts, are similar among themselves. They identify with each other. That's what convinced me that I had a problem.

That four-day treatment turned into a recommendation for three months. It was a week of inpatient to withdraw, then it was a halfway house with a campus, so a partial hospitalization-type program. The counselors held meetings and kept real close track of you with drug testing. You met with a group led by professional counselors once a week and had sessions with the physician once a month. The whole program is designed to slowly get people to the point of discharge and safe return to a medical practice.

I shared a two-bedroom apartment with four grown men, trying to cook for themselves, shop, and wash. [*Laugh*] They're all detoxing. It's funny when you're sitting on the porch in recovery with people who understand you, it's very comfortable, and so you're able to see the truth. You're no longer in denial. It was an environment where people could reorient your thinking, not by virtue of pointing out the truth or educating you, but just by living it.

To return home, you have to establish a safe place to go and then spend a weekend there first. You have to find a sponsor, somebody who's been there and done that and has agreed to work through all the AA steps with you. You also have to read the Alcoholics Anonymous book that was written in the thirties and is still the mainstay of the 12-step program. You work through the book with a sponsor, do all the steps, and you have to do an inventory.

You examine your life through sober eyes and see what was amiss in your thinking and behaving and character. They talk in the AA book about addiction being like an obsession of the mind. When your thoughts race up, you need to go get messed up; you need that drink. Then once the alcoholic starts drinking, they can't control the amount because they just wanna go to the bitter end until they get that feeling, that sigh of relief. You think, "I'm gonna be okay and maybe one more drink won't hurt," and then it on takes a life of its own. It's a mental illness, a kind of an internal brain disease.

Then I found my sponsor, someone who had been there two years before and was returning for a five-day revisit. This guy lived in my town, had a job, a family, and all his drug tests were negative. He'd done the Healthcare Professional Recovery Program, a state mandated monitoring program so the center knew he was good. His story was that he'd had 92 felonies, lost his license, was using 120 Vicodin a day and had been totally messed up, way worse than me. He said, "I finally got my feet on the ground. I got my license back, I got a job, my wife and I worked it out, we have a home together." That was a light for me, hearing his story. I asked him to be my sponsor, so we started comparing notes. He'd grown up, probably within miles of me, and we went to the same high school, college, and medical school. And it turns out that his office was two miles from my clinic!

So I set up a weekend at home. I was going to stay at my brother's house, my 'safe space' and meet with my sponsor. Then my brother called saying he couldn't be home that weekend but his friend Ed would be there. And the day before I was to leave, I let it slip that my brother would be away and the counselors said, "You're about to get on a plane tomorrow and the night before you're telling us this. Don't you see the deceit here and the problem. Isn't Ed a drug user?" So, they revoked my discharge.

And then divorce papers got served. Suddenly I had nothing. All the money was gone with the divorce. I didn't have a car. I didn't have clothes. My credit cards were chopped up because they were not being paid. I was homeless, penniless, jobless, and pretty desperate. So my three month program turned into five months and three weeks.

But at least I had a sponsor when I was discharged. I wasn't drinking, I wasn't drugging. I had a way to deal with the world that that didn't involve drinking and taking a drug. It was actually a very valuable lesson.

That very first year of being sober, my sponsor said, "You gotta go to this IDAA (International Doctors in Alcoholics Anonymous) annual meeting. It's like Cadu (Caduceus meetings for recovering medical professionals)." And at that time I was pretty destitute, but I managed to scrap enough money to take my oldest daughter, she was 14.

IDAA has an Alateen group for teenagers where they learn about alcoholism from each other. And they were the only kids my daughter had met who had a drunken doctor dad. They're like, "Oh my God, your dad was that up!" "Oh, mine was worse!" "Do you know what it was like not to be able to bring my friends home?" "One day he's brilliant and nice and one day he's a raving maniac." They even have a Betty Ford-designed program for the younger kids, so even seven-year-olds can understand what their parents are doing and meet other kids growing up with this. They learn the difference between the diseased alcoholic behavior and the real father they love, so the kids get engaged in recovery. My two youngest ones started when they were very young. And when she turned 20, my oldest daughter didn't wanna graduate from the Alateen; that's where she met her best friends. So she started Al20, her own little subsection of AA.

I did go back to work in my hospital clinic when I left the treatment center. The medical side of the clinic was being handled by somebody else, but I was still doing the business part. I was really good at business, so the clinic became wildly successful. I could also manage the medical stuff because it was a narrow spectrum of medicine. It was musculoskeletal, toxicology, safety ergonomics—stuff that I could learn every detail of. It's like ophthalmology, right, just knowing eyeballs; not a lot of mystery! [*Laugh*]

My life from then on was pretty smooth. I had one bump in the road with a relationship that went bad, and I suffered a year of depression and regret, but I never drank. And eventually, years later, I met somebody else, and we've been married for 20 years and have a beautiful blended family and grandkids. My wife is in Al-Anon. AA added Al-Anon to help people affected by alcoholics; it could be your parent, kids, spouse, sibling; anybody whose life is entwined with yours and is watching powerless. She was married to a cocaine, alcohol addicted ophthalmologist so she understands the whole recovery thing. She'd tolerated the intolerable and tried to make excuses for him and help him be normal, even though that's impossible. If you're living with an active alcoholic, you can't control them and you can't fix the problem because you didn't cause it. But if you sit there for years trying to do these things, you get sick.

So, with a recovering alcoholic and a partner in Al-Anon, it's kind of like a blessed marriage, because there's you and her and you each have your own higher power, which is something greater than yourself, helping you to live a sane life. Your craziness doesn't go away, but with recovery, you learn to check it out. If I've got big decisions to make, I know I'd better call somebody to ask for help because I can't trust my thinking all the time. Initially, that would be true a lot of the time, eventually it became true just some of the time, and later it became rare to get that sick thinking that I needed to go get drunk. But it comes up still.

Obviously, life is not all roses, but the joy overwhelms the problems. I retired this year, so I get to travel around the country, visit the kids. I've started to go to yoga every day. My body feels good and my brain feels good and we're both joyous. I can forgive myself for how I used to be because I was sick. And if I could have done it differently, I would've done it differently, but I wasn't able to. But you know, I can forgive myself.

---

### Discussion or Writing Prompts

1 Are you able to feel empathy for Dr Benson's story? Does the fact that he experienced childhood trauma, had a family history of addiction, and was pressured to be a doctor make a difference?

2 "Alcoholism was not really considered a disease; it was treated like a moral deficiency." What were the prevailing attitudes about Alcohol and Substance Use Disorders in medical school or training? What are your attitudes?

3 Dr Benson was able to get through his medical school and training without being held accountable because he was scoring well on his tests. How could someone like him be held accountable? What should be the clues?

4 How you think Dr Benson was able to turn the corner? What aspects of his treatment or recovery or life situation seem most relevant?

5 "If I've got big decisions to make, I know I'd better call somebody to ask for help because I can't trust my thinking all the time." Why is asking for help critical for someone with a substance use disorder? How about for people without an addiction?

6 Examine the difference between forgiving yourself and avoiding necessary accountability. When does self-forgiveness make it more likely that you will hold yourself accountable rather than blaming others for your problems?

---

### Resources

International Doctors in Alcoholics Anonymous. (n.d.). https://www.idaa. org/.

Alcoholics Anonymous. (n.d.). https://www.aa.org/.

National Institute on Alcohol Abuse and Alcoholism. (n.d.). https://alcoholtreatment.niaaa.nih.gov/.

# Bibliography

## Vulnerability, Perfectionism

Brown, B. (2012). *Daring Greatly*. Gotham Books.

Johnson, K. M., Slavin, S. J., & Takahashi, T. A. (2023). Excellent vs excessive: Helping trainees balance performance and perfectionism. *Journal of Graduate Medical Education, 15*(4), 424–427. https://doi.org/10.4300/JGME-D-23-00003.1

Norman, K. (December 2020). Overcoming the trauma of making a medical error: Self-forgiveness is an important skill for recovery. *Journal of Urgent Care Medicine*, 9–11. https://www.jucm.com/wp-content/uploads/2021/02/2020-1539-11-Perspectives.pdf

Harbach, C. (2011). *The Art of Fielding*. Little, Brown and Company.


## Depression/Anxiety

Depression and Bipolar Support Alliance. (n.d.). https://www.dbsalliance.org/

Anxiety and Depression Association of America. (n.d.). Understanding anxiety. https://adaa.org/Understanding-Anxiety

Jain, N., & Stonnington, C. (2024). Physician and medical student mental health. In R Boland and M Verduin (Eds.), *Kaplan and Sadock's Comprehensive Textbook of Psychiatry* (11th ed., chap. 30.8).

Nesse, R. (2020). *Good Reasons for Bad Feelings: Insights from the Frontier of Evolutionary Psychiatry*. Penguin.

Styron, W. (1990). *Darkness Visible*. Vintage.


## Suicide

American Foundation for Suicide Prevention. (n.d.). Support after suicide loss for healthcare professionals and organizations. https://afsp.org/support-after-suicide-loss-for-healthcare-professionals-and-organizations/

American Medical Association. (n.d.). AMA STEPS Forward: After Physician Suicide toolkit. https://edhub.ama-assn.org/steps-forward/module/2813039

## Licensure/Credentialing

Dyrbye, L. N., West, C. P., Sinsky, C. A., Goeders, L. E., Satele, D. V., & Shanafelt, T. D. (2017). Medical licensure questions and physician reluctance to seek care for mental health conditions. *Mayo Clinic Proceedings, 92*(10), 1486–1493. https://doi.org/10.1016/j.mayocp.2017.06.020

Dr. Lorna Breen Heroes Foundation. (n.d.). Improving licensure & credentialing applications. https://drlornabreen.org/removebarriers/

## Addiction

Geyer, H. (2023). *Ending the crisis: Mayo Clinic's guide to opioid addiction and safe opioid use.* Mayo Clinic Press.

Merlo, L. J., Campbell, M. D., Shea, C., White, W., Skipper, G. E., Sutton, J. A., & DuPont, R. L. (2022). Essential components of physician health program monitoring for substance use disorder: A survey of participants 5 years post successful program completion. *The American Journal on Addictions, 31*(2), 115–122.

Hill, A. B. (2017). Breaking the stigma — A physician's perspective on self-care and recovery. *New England Journal of Medicine, 376*, 1103–1105. https://doi.org/10.1056/NEJMp1615974

Oreskovich, M. R., Shanafelt, T., Dyrbye, L. N., Tan, L., Sotile, W., Satele, D., West, C. P., Sloan, J., & Boone, S. (2015). The prevalence of substance use disorders in American physicians. *The American Journal on Addictions, 24*(1), 30–38. https://doi.org/10.1111/ajad.12173

Kingsolver, B. (2020). *Demon Copperhead.* HarperCollins Publishers.

International Doctors in Alcoholics Anonymous. (n.d.). https://www.idaa.org/

Alcoholics Anonymous. (n.d.). https://www.aa.org/

National Institute on Alcohol Abuse and Alcoholism. (n.d.). https://alcoholtreatment.niaaa.nih.gov/

## Peer Support/Relationships

American Medical Association. (n.d.). Peer support programs for physicians: Mitigate the effects of emotional stressors through peer support. *AMA STEPS Forward.* https://edhub.ama-assn.org/steps-forward/module/2767766

Finney, R. E., Jacob, A., Johnson, J., Mesner, H., Pulos, B., & Sviggum, H. (2021). Implementation of a second victim peer support program in a large anesthesia department. *American Association of Nurse Anesthetists Journal, 89*, 235–244.

Brown, B. [Brené Brown]. (2010, December 10). Brené Brown on Empathy [Video]. YouTube. https://www.youtube.com/watch?v=1Evwgu369Jw

Balint, M. (1955). The doctor, his patient, and the illness. *The Lancet, 265*(6866), 683–688. https://doi.org/10.1016/S0140-6736(55)91061-8

American Balint Society. (n.d.). https://americanbalintsociety.org/

The Schwartz Center for Compassionate Healthcare. (n.d.). Schwartz rounds. https://www.theschwartzcenter.org/programs/schwartz-rounds/

Toll, E. T., & Sinsky, C. A. (2023). The deep work of doctoring—Prioritizing relationships in medicine. *JAMA Internal Medicine, 183*(9), 904–905. https://doi.org/10.1001/jamainternmed.2023.3012

Shem, S. (1978). *The House of God.* Berkley Publishing Group.

## Burnout/Well-Being/COVID-19

National Academies of Sciences, Engineering, and Medicine. (2019). *Taking Action against Clinician Burnout: A Systems Approach to Professional Well-Being*. The National Academies Press.

Perlo, J., Balik, B., Swensen, S., Kabcenell, A., Landsman, J., & Feeley, D. (2017). *IHI Framework for Improving Joy in Work*. Institute for Healthcare Improvement.

U.S. Department of Health and Human Services. (2022). *Promoting Emotional Well-Being and Mental Health in the Workplace [PDF file]*. https://www.hhs.gov/sites/default/files/workplace-mental-health-well-being.pdf

Agata, S., Grzegorz, W., Ilona, B., Violetta, K., & Katarzyna, S. (2023). Prevalence of burnout among healthcare professionals during the COVID-19 pandemic and associated factors—A scoping review. *International Journal of Occupational Medicine and Environmental Health, 36*(1), 21–58. https://doi.org/10.13075/ijomeh.1896.02007

Shanafelt, T., Ripp, J., & Trockel, M. (2020). Understanding and addressing sources of anxiety among health care professionals during the COVID-19 pandemic. *JAMA, 323*(21), 2133–2134. https://doi.org/10.1001/jama.2020.5893

Shanafelt, T. D., & Noseworthy, J. H. (2017). Executive leadership and physician well-being: Nine organizational strategies to promote engagement and reduce burnout. *Mayo Clinic Proceedings, 92*(1), 129–146. https://doi.org/10.1016/j.mayocp.2016.10.004

Mete, M., Goldman, C., Shanafelt, T., & Marchalik, D. (2022). Impact of leadership behavior on physician well-being, burnout, professional fulfillment, and intent to leave: A multicenter cross-sectional survey study. *BMJ Open, 12*(6), e057554. https://doi.org/10.1136/bmjopen-2021-057554

Gold, J. (2024). *How Do You Feel? One Doctor's Search for Humanity in Medicine*. Simon & Schuster.

## Resilience

Southwick, S. M., & Charney, D. S. (2018). *Resilience: The Science of Mastering Life's Greatest Challenges*. Cambridge University Press.

Shankar, M. (2023, June 15). Preparatory Division Commencement Address 2023 [Video]. YouTube. https://www.youtube.com/watch?v=iSii6pIDQCM

## Humanities

Association of American Medical Colleges. (n.d.). The fundamental role of the arts and humanities in medical education. https://store.aamc.org/downloadable/download/sample/sample_id/382/

## Boundaries

AMA- Code. (n.d.). Breach of security in electronic medical records. https://www.ama-assn.org/breach-security-electronic-medical-records

Association of American Medical Colleges. (n.d.). Healthy boundary setting in order to maintain wellness. https://www.aamc.org/media/60651/download

Herbst, R., Sump, C., & Riddle, S. (2023) Staying in bounds: A framework for setting workplace boundaries to promote physician wellness. *Journal of Hospital Medicine, 18*(12), 1139–1143. https://shmpublications.onlinelibrary.wiley.com/doi/full/10.1002/jhm.13102

## Mistreatment/Microaggressions

American Medical Association. (n.d.). Bullying in the health care workplace: A guide to prevention & mitigation. *AMA*. https://www.ama-assn.org/practice-management/physician-health/bullying-health-care-workplace-guide-prevention-mitigation#:~:text=The%20AMA%20defines%20workplace%20bullying%20as%20repeated%2C%20emotionally,embarrass%2C%20undermine%2C%20threaten%2C%20or%20otherwise%20harm%20the%20target

Bajaj, S. S., Tu, L., & Stanford, F. C. (2021). Superhuman, but never enough: Black women in medicine. *The Lancet, 398*(10309), 1398–1399. https://doi.org/10.1016/S0140-6736(21)02217-0

Ehie, O., Muse, I., Hill, L., & Bastien, A. (2021). Professionalism: Microaggression in the healthcare setting. *Current Opinion in Anesthesiology, 34*(2), 131–136. https://www.ncbi.nlm.nih.gov/pmc/articles/PMC7984763/

Fabi, R., & Johnson, L. S. M. (2024). Responding effectively to disruptive patient behaviors: Beyond behavior contracts. *JAMA, 331*(10), 823–824. https://doi.org/10.1001/jama.2024.0216

Lerner, H. (2002). *The Dance of Connection: How to Talk to Someone When You're Mad, Hurt, Scared, Frustrated, Insulted, Betrayed, or Desperate.* William Morrow Paperbacks.

Rowe, S. G., Stewart, M. T., Van Horne, S., Pierre, C., Wang, H., Manukyan, M., Bair-Merritt, M., Lee-Parritz, A., Rowe, M. P., Shanafelt, T., & Trockel, M. (2022). Mistreatment experiences, protective workplace systems, and occupational distress in physicians. *JAMA Network Open, 5*(5), e2210768. https://doi.org/10.1001/jamanetworkopen.2022.10768

## Family/Reproductive Planning

Bakkensen, J. B., Smith, K. S., Cheung, E. O., Moreno, P. I., Goldman, K. N., Lawson, A. K., & Feinberg, E. C. (2023). Childbearing, infertility, and career trajectories among women in medicine. *JAMA Network Open, 6*(7), e2326192. https://doi.org/10.1001/jamanetworkopen.2023.26192

Jakubowski, J. S., Baltzer, H., Lipa, J. E., & Snell, L. (2023). Parental-leave policies and perceptions of pregnancy during surgical residency training in North America: A scoping review. *Canadian Journal of Surgery, 66*(2), E132–E138. https://doi.org/10.1503/cjs.009321

Johnson, K., Posner, S. F., Biermann, J., Cordero, J. F., Atrash, H. K., Parker, C. S., Boulet, S., & Curtis, M. G. (2006). Recommendations to improve preconception health and health care--United States. A report of the CDC/ATSDR Preconception Care Work Group and the Select Panel on Preconception Care. *MMWR Recommendations and Reports, 55*(RR-6), 1–23.

## Professional Identity/Role-Models

Benbassat, J. (2014). Role modeling in medical education: The importance of a reflective imitation. *Academic Medicine, 89*(4), 550–554. https://doi.org/10.1097/ACM.0000000000000189

Cruess, R. L., Cruess, S. R., Boudreau, J. D., Snell, L., & Steinert, Y. (2015). A schematic representation of the professional identity formation and socialization of medical students and residents: A guide for medical educators. *Academic Medicine, 90*(6), 718–725. https://doi.org/10.1097/ACM.0000000000000700

## Delivering bad news

American Academy of Family Physicians. (2001). Breaking bad news. *American Family Physician.* https://www.aafp.org/pubs/afp/issues/2001/1215/p1975.html

Association of American Medical Colleges. (n.d.). Delivering grave news with empathy and honesty. https://www.aamc.org/news/delivering-grave-news-empathy-and-honesty

Kalanithi, P. (2016). *When Breath Becomes Air.* Random House.

## Integrative Medicine

Mayo Clinic. (n.d.). Integrative medicine and health – Overview. https://www.mayoclinic.org/tests-procedures/complementary-alternative-medicine/about/pac-20393581

# Index

Printed in the United States
by Baker & Taylor Publisher Services

Printed in the United States
by Baker & Taylor Publisher Services